HEALTH CARE REFORM
AND
AMERICAN POLITICS

WHAT EVERYONE NEEDS TO KNOW®

HEALTH CARE REFORM
AND
AMERICAN POLITICS

WHAT EVERYONE NEEDS TO KNOW®

3rd EDITION

LAWRENCE R. JACOBS
AND
THEDA SKOCPOL

OXFORD
UNIVERSITY PRESS

Oxford University Press is a department of the University of Oxford.
It furthers the University's objective of excellence in research,
scholarship, and education by publishing worldwide. Oxford is a
registered trademark of Oxford University Press
in the UK and certain other countries.

Published in the United States of America by Oxford University Press
198 Madison Avenue, New York, NY 10016, United States of America

Library of Congress Cataloging-in-Publication Data
is available

ISBN 978-0-19-026203-7 (hbk.)
ISBN 978-0-19-026204-4 (pbk.)

"What Everyone Needs to Know" is a registered
trademark of Oxford University Press.

1 3 5 7 9 8 6 4 2
Printed in the United States of America
on acid-free paper

CONTENTS

PREFACE AND ACKNOWLEDGMENTS

On March 23, 2010, President Barack Obama signed into law a landmark in U.S. social legislation, the Patient Protection and Affordable Care Act. In the two weeks before the critical vote on the first day of spring, and especially in the hours before, the two authors of this book were e-mailing back and forth furiously. Would the President and House Speaker Nancy Pelosi manage to cobble together enough votes from House Democrats to pass comprehensive health reform? Would quarrels over abortion derail the deal at the last minute? Which provisions—spelling out who would benefit, and who would pay—would remain in the bill at the end?

Our interest was intense not just because the outcome was uncertain until almost the last minute, but also because both of us, Larry Jacobs and Theda Skocpol, have been fascinated by the politics of health care reform for many years. We have written about past battles—for Medicare, for Clinton's failed Health Security reform—and we have thought about what successes and failures in social-policy battles mean for American politics. Even before Obama's White House signaled in early 2009 that it would proceed with a gargantuan effort to get Congress to pass comprehensive health reform amidst partisan polarization, the Great Recession, and intense special interest lobbying, the two of us had geared up to look at health care issues in the Obama presidency. After all, this was a

Democratic President who came to office, along with large Democratic Congressional majorities, at a time when the U.S. health care system was clearly broken—facing skyrocketing costs and receding coverage of health care for middle-class and lower-income families. Obama and other Democrats had promised to act on much-needed reforms. Would they try to keep their promise, even after the economic crises intensified and Republicans signaled total opposition? Would they succeed, or fall short as so many would-be reformers before them had done? It was bound to be a fascinating political story that would tell us a lot about what is possible, and not, in U.S. politics in the early twenty-first century.

We were able to finish the first edition of this book just a few months after President Obama's signing ceremony, because we closely studied the process of health reform through all of its phases. From 2007 on, we tracked media coverage, public opinion, health-care trends, and statements by politicians and organized groups; during 2009 and early 2010, we went to Washington, DC, to interview key players in Congress and the White House. As we gathered real-time facts and perceptions, we could draw upon the best analyses in political science— about public opinion, about patterns of Congressional decision making and voting, about lobbyists and socvial movements, and about the effect of institutional rules and previous public policies on current debates. Our immersion in currently unfolding events, while armed with powerful social-science tools, put us in a position to analyze what was happening promptly. We moved equally quickly after the Supreme Court upheld Affordable Care on June 28, 2012.

Our experience as historically and institutionally oriented political scientists also enables us to think about what comes next in health reform after the laws are on the books and affirmed by the Supreme Court, as administrators, politicians, and interest groups struggle about how to put them into effect or revise them. We have aimed to pinpoint the next struggles in health reform, to share our insights about unfolding developments with fellow citizens and with students and observers who care about the future of health care reform. That is why we put in the effort to finish this book and get it into the public sphere by the early fall of 2010, before the first national election after the enactment of Affordable Care. This new edition allows us to extend our analysis through the intense legal and electoral battles in 2012.

Many have helped us get it done. David McBride at Oxford University Press saw the potential and supported our effort to move quickly, as did Alexandra Dauler. Invaluable and highly skilled research assistance was provided by Melanie Burns, Charles Gregory, and Patrick Carter at the University of Minnesota, and by Vanessa Williamson at Harvard University (who not only worked on several chapters but also prepared the time line and glossary for this book). Larry Jacobs appreciates support from the University of Minnesota, one of the country's original land-grant public universities, and from the Hubert H. Humphrey School of Public Affairs. We are grateful to the Russell Sage Foundation and its President Eric Wanner for its support of a scholarly working group on "Obama's Agenda and the Dynamics of U.S. Politics." The two of us are coordinating this working group, and our research on health reform is, in part, supported by the Foundation's grant. We benefited from discussions with other members of the group, each of whom is tracking a policy area of his or her own. We also want to acknowledge the support of the Robert Wood Johnson Foundation that allowed us to track health reform after its enactment in 2010. Finally, we thank our spouses, Julie Schumacher and Bill Skocpol. Bill, as he always does with Theda's books, read through the final manuscript and made suggestions to improve clarity. Both Julie and Bill put up with their partner spending almost all the time for weeks on the challenging and fascinating task of finishing this book.

Lawrence Jacobs, St. Paul, Minnesota
Theda Skocpol, Cambridge, Massachusetts

INTRODUCTION: A TURNING POINT FOR U.S. HEALTH CARE AND POLITICS

On Tuesday, March 23, 2010, several hundred people crowded into the East Room of the White House to witness President Barack Obama sign into law the Patient Protection and Affordable Care Act. The mood was exultant, and the President was interrupted "repeatedly with cheers, applause and standing ovations" from more than 200 House and Senate members joined by Victoria Reggae Kennedy, widow of the late Massachusetts Senator and life-long health-reform crusader Ted Kennedy, as well as by regular citizens who had experienced first-hand the travails of the nation's patchwork system of health care coverage.[1] Standing close, and wearing an electric blue tie just like the President's, was eleven-year-old Marcelas Owens of Seattle, "who became an advocate for health reform after his mother died without insurance"; also watching was Connie Anderson, "whose sister is Natoma Canfield, the Ohio cancer patient whose struggles to pay for rising health premiums became a case in point for Mr. Obama."[2]

In the President's words on that Tuesday in the East Room, "the bill I'm signing will set in motion reforms that generations of Americans have fought for and marched for and hungered to see," enshrining "the core principle that everybody should have some basic security when it comes to their health care." Over the course of the past century, modern health care has become increasingly effective at saving and improving lives—and also steadily more expensive for individuals, businesses, and governments. Because people value health and life so much, they do all they can to pay the price for care, and can even go bankrupt in the process.[3] The U.S. health-care financing system in existence before the current health reform law was enacted relied on partial government programs and patchwork private-market arrangements to protect many citizens, but far from all of them.

In the United States as of the early 21st century, working-aged men and women and their children were not assured of health insurance coverage. Businesses need healthy workers and many of them struggled to pay rising insurance premiums to cover their employees, often to the detriment of a business's ability to compete on international markets against firms in other countries where government assures health coverage. Other U.S. businesses, especially small firms, just have not been able to afford to even try to pay for insurance for their employees and their families. In an economy where some employers offer health insurance and others do not, many Americans struggled to get a job with benefits and then hold onto it for dear life, quite literally, even if it would make more sense to move to a new career or a new community in a better job. The more attractive job was not worth it if it did not offer health coverage. Private health insurance companies in the United States have grown into industry giants arranging coverage in negotiations with big employers on the one side, and hospitals and doctors, on the other side. But insurance companies have strong incentives to protect their profit margins by dumping people who get costly illnesses, such as cancer, something they could do before the current reforms were enacted. They also hiked rates with little scrutiny and avoided offering coverage to segments of the population, occupational groups, or parts of the country likely to have high health costs.

As modern health care has improved and increased in cost, reformers in the United States have repeatedly tried to use the regulatory and financial powers of democratic government to help citizens defray medical costs and gain access to quality care. The quest started all the way back in the 1910s during the Bull-Moose presidential campaign of Teddy Roosevelt and state-level campaigns of the American Association for Labor Legislation; it continued through the New Deal and the drive of President Harry Truman for "compulsory health insurance" at the end of World War II; and it sputtered on through subsequent efforts during the presidencies of John Kennedy, Richard Nixon, Jimmy Carter, and, most recently, Bill Clinton, who, in 1993–1994, called for "health care that's always there, health care that can never be taken away." Universal health care was established in one way or another in every other industrial or industrializing nation. But in the United States, health care reformers (as advocates of universal coverage are labeled) have run into bitter political opposition and, every time prior to 2010, fallen short of achieving guaranteed coverage for all citizens. The best reformers could do, in major steps toward this goal, came decades ago, in the mid-1960s, when Medicare was enacted to help cover physician and hospital costs for the elderly and Medicaid was enacted to pay for care for some of the very poor.

The century-long Sisyphean effort by American advocates of universal health insurance, to push that weighty boulder up the mountain, explains why, after the rock finally tipped over the top in March 2010, Vice President Joe Biden was picked up on a super-sensitive microphone at the signing ceremony exclaiming—sotto-voce—that it was "a big f…ing deal." This turned out to be one of Biden's trademark loveable gaffes, soon to be propagated on YouTube and printed on T-shirts. Indeed, in the assessment of many pundits, the new Affordable Care Act of 2010 instantly took its place as a landmark in U.S. social legislation, comparable to Social Security legislation enacted in 1935, Civil Rights legislation enacted in 1964, and, of course, Medicare.

The tortuous path to comprehensive health reform did not come to an end in March 2010. Like a suspense movie where the apparent climatic scene merely sets up even more hair-raising plot twists, the November 2010 elections swept Tea Party conservatives into Washington and state capitals who were devoted to the full repeal of reform. That was not all. Twenty-six states mounted determined legal efforts to have Affordable Care declared unconstitutional. The momentous June 2012 Supreme Court decision to uphold the law by a narrow majority was followed three years later, in June 2015, by yet another pivotal high court decision preserving major parts of the health reform law. Together, these Supreme Court rulings ensure the legislation's survival over the long run, even as partisan battles and court challenges of particular regulations and expenditures continue. The arc of American history now bends toward health care for all—and greater efficiency in the system as a whole.

What does health reform actually do? Affordable Care promises key changes in a complex, expensive, and fragmented set of U.S. arrangements for paying for health care.[4] Especially notable are popular new benefits:

- For at least twenty-six million Americans who previously lacked insurance, the new law expands access to Medicaid (the federal-state insurance program for low-income people) and provides subsidies to help small businesses and individuals with modest incomes purchase reasonably priced private insurance plans on state-run marketplaces called "exchanges." Nearly 12 million gained coverage in the initial two years of exchange operations. Following the June 2012 Supreme Court ruling, states had the option of whether to expand Medicaid, but generous funding and pressure from hospitals and citizens has persuaded 30 blue and red states to proceed, and more states are likely to follow suit before long.
- For older people on Medicare, the new law is delivering free preventive checkups and more complete subsidies for prescription drug coverage.
- For individual purchasers as well as some 151 million Americans who already have health insurance via their employers, the new law includes key regulatory protections.[5] Private insurers can no longer avoid or cut people

with serious "preexisting" health problems. They must also allow young adults to remain on parental insurance plans until age 26—a step that has already extended health coverage to 2.3 million young adults, allowing three-quarters of them to become insured.[6]

Beyond these subsidies and protections for ordinary people currently with or without health insurance, the new law addresses several longstanding, daunting problems—rising economic inequalities and total national health care costs. About 80 percent of new benefits promised by the Affordable Care Act go to lower and middle-income Americans—the people whose employers do not provide health insurance, yet who are not poor or old enough for existing federal programs, and these expanded benefits are slated to be paid for primarily by higher taxes on wealthier citizens and by fees assessed on parts of the health care industry.[7] This is why *New York Times* columnist David Leonhardt calls Affordable Care "the federal government's biggest attack on economic inequality" since the late 1970s, when incomes for the well-to-do started skyrocketing even as wages and benefits for ordinary Americans entered a prolonged period of stagnation or decline.[8]

In addition, the nation's overall- health care bill has stopped rising at a breakneck pace. After increasing at rates as high as 16 percent during 1980s and nearly double digits through 1990s, the "health inflation" rate has slowed to 3–4 percent (the lowest rate of increase in half a century) and that stodgy nonpartisan score keeper the Congressional Budget Office has lowered its initial projections for growth in health care costs.[9]

The new law requires virtually all Americans to buy basic health insurance coverage, just as all drivers are required to have accident insurance. Backed up by subsidies to render health insurance affordable for lower-and middle-income people, this "individual mandate" is designed to make sure that people do not wait until they or a loved one becomes ill, getting the healthy into the system from the start. The law also includes eventual taxes on very expensive private insurance plans, intended to make them less prevalent, along with incentives for more efficient payments to physicians and hospitals, intended to move the nation toward paying for results in health care, rather than for sheer numbers of tests and procedures.

Both President Obama and key Democratic leaders in the Senate and House touted the long-term deficit-reduction features of this legislation. Their claim, borne out by the evidence so far, is that expanded coverage and cost control go together. Emergency-room care for uninsured people can be more expensive than the preventive care available to the insured. Moreover, by making it impossible for insurance companies to profit by cutting or avoiding sick people, the law is starting to encourage insurers to make profits by promoting greater health care efficiency. Under the Affordable Care Act, rules for the U.S. health insurance system are more like those in the National Football League—where teams have an incentive to hire, pay, and draft smart under a cap—than like those in major league baseball, where anything goes and the Yankees and a couple of other teams that can afford to spend the most millions usually win, while poor teams just get worse and the middle-of-the-pack spenders fall short of the top.

A TOUGH BATTLE

Joyful as the celebration was at the signing of the Affordable Care Act, there was also an undertone of exhaustion in the room. Only Democrats were to be found among the 200 or so lawmakers in attendance on March 23, 2010—despite the fact that months had been spent trying to woo Republican moderates who, in principle, agreed that the nation's health insurance system needed major fixes. Many longstanding Republican ideas about health care reform were embodied in the bills finally enacted, with tight margins, by Democrats alone in the House and Senate. In fact, the new Affordable Care framework closely resembles the approach enacted for the state of Massachusetts under the governorship of Republican Mitt

Romney.[10] But Republicans themselves, even those who contributed ideas to the bills, refused to vote for or argue on behalf of the 2010 federal reform. Indeed, Republicans in the Senate refused even to let measures proceed to final debate in regular order, using their minority of 41 votes in the final weeks to prevent majority decisions in that chamber.

Bitter partisan opposition erupted repeatedly from spring 2009 to spring 2010, at each of the many steps it took to get health reform bills through three House committees plus the full House of Representatives, as well as through two Senate committees and the full Senate. Partisanship meant that a process always sure to be tricky ended up taking months more than originally envisaged by the President and the media. Even if many Democrats and some Republicans had been able to cooperate in Congress, there would have been prolonged debates, as every major industry and interest group in the country weighed in on changes in which all have a stake. But the inevitable complexity turned into a bitter and dramatic story full of twists and turns worthy of a Hollywood thriller or a complex detective novel. Reform was repeatedly declared dead, only to live on, if barely at times, over the first fifteen months of Barack Obama's presidency.

Obama's signature on legislation promising comprehensive health reform was a crucial turning point, but it was far from the end of the story. The Affordable Care Act of 2010 simply created a framework and a timetable, and its many subsidies and regulations were implemented gradually. Some provisions went into effect by the summer and fall of 2010, such as rules to help children and young adults get insurance coverage, payments to help elderly Americans cover high costs for prescription drugs, and subsidies to help very ill people afford insurance. But the most important provisions were phased in starting in 2014. Both the federal government and all fifty states took many steps to carry out new rules and extend tax breaks and subsidies to businesses and citizens.

None of this has happened in an atmosphere of political calm or good will. After the March 2010 signing in the White

House, conservative officials in twenty-six states, mostly Republicans, filed lawsuits asking the federal courts to reverse all or parts of what they derisively called "ObamaCare." After the Supreme Court rejected their case in June 2012, conservatives were not done with the courts. Their next legal assault aimed at stripping away subsidies that over 6 million Americans relied upon to purchase insurance. It too reached the Supreme Court in 2015 before being rejected.

Meanwhile, health insurers and businesses organized lobbying efforts in Congress and state legislatures to influence federal and state administrators who wrote rules to carry insurance reforms into full effect. Business interests and conservative groups raised money and mobilized voters to elect more Republicans to Congress between 2010 and 2014, in the hope of reversing health reform, starving it for funds, or enacting important changes in taxes and regulations. As the Affordable Care Act has taken full effect, it profoundly changes politics in voting booths, courts, legislatures, and bureaucracies. How much of the full plan is ultimately realized will depend on future policy decisions and unfolding political battles.

WHAT HAPPENED AND WHAT IT MEANS

This book, therefore, tells two intertwined stories: the story of the new U.S. health care policies fashioned in 2009 and 2010, and the story of the past and future political battles about reform. Every American has a stake in understanding the health care issues and the political questions at stake in this momentous reform effort. The story is a dramatic one, and we plan to tell it in the coming chapters as concisely, vividly, and understandably as possible. As scholars, we adhere to the best standards of truth in our craft; the footnotes spell out sources for each of our major factual claims and cite quotes or interviews. We are also American citizens who care about making sense to our fellow citizens; and we love a good narrative.

The chapters that come answer the following questions—
with the overall flow from chapter to chapter following the
time line laid out at the end of this introduction.

- Why was the time ripe after the 2008 election for another
  push for big health reforms? Back in 1993 and 1994, a
  previous Democratic President and Congress had come
  to grief attempting comprehensive reforms, so why did
  the next Democratic President and Congress decide to
  try again? Chapter 1 answers this question.
- Why did the drama unfold as it did during 2009, the critical year in which both houses of Congress fashioned
  health reform bills? How did an initially broad consensus
  that a broken health insurance system needed fixing
  devolve into bitter, partisan struggles that left only Democrats willing to move forward with reform legislation—
  even though many Republican ideas were incorporated
  into the reform bills? Chapter 2 tackles these questions—
  and it is quite a story.
- In mid-January 2010, when Republican and (at that point)
  Tea-Party darling Scott Brown shockingly won the
  Massachusetts Senate seat formerly held by Ted Kennedy, it
  suddenly looked as if health reform was dead. No matter
  that a year had been spent and bills had already passed the
  House and Senate; Republicans in the Senate now had 41
  votes they could use to filibuster final legislation. In one of
  the most dramatic twists of the health reform odyssey,
  President Obama and House and Senate leaders turned
  what seemed like defeat into an even bolder version of health
  reform than the bills on the table at the end of 2009. How did
  that happen? Chapter 3 analyzes the final twists and turns in
  the amazing endgame of health reform legislation.
- What did all that *Sturm und Drang* actually produce for
  Americans in different circumstances, for the national
  economy, and for the national budgetary situation?
  Chapter 4 spells it out, taking into account the Supreme
  Court's historic rulings in June 2012 and June 2015 to

uphold most of the law. If the law is ultimately implemented as intended, the vast majority of Americans will
benefit, with the wealthy and certain businesses paying
most of the tab. Most employers and workers will gain
from a more level playing field and from economic
growth spurred by successful health reform. If the Act's
provisions to control cost increases work as intended, the
federal budget deficit will shrink, not grow.

• But "it ain't over yet." Writing and enacting comprehensive health reform legislation is one thing; putting it all
into effect in an angry political climate is another. How
are federal and state officials working to implement the
new rules, subsidies, and taxes—and what kind of pushback are they getting from lobbyists representing powerful economic interests? How has the passage of health
reform sparked recrimination by Republicans who appeal
to citizen anxieties about health reform, even as Democrats
point to valuable benefits for young people, small businesses, seniors, and middle-Americans? How have these
battles changed now that new benefits are reaching
millions of people (Democrats and Republicans alike)
and the Supreme Court has twice upheld Affordable
Care. Chapter 5 offers a comprehensive road map to the
ongoing issues and struggles.

TIMELINE OF HEALTH REFORM EVENTS

March 24, 2007   Only weeks into his presidential bid, Obama performs unevenly at a health care forum with other presidential candidates. He remarks, "I will judge my first term as president based on...whether we have delivered the kind of health care that every American deserves and that our system can afford."[1]

August 28, 2008   Senator Obama accepts the Democratic nomination in Denver, CO. In his speech he says, "Now is the time to finally keep the promise of affordable, accessible health care for every single American."[2]

February 17, 2009   The President signs the American Recovery and Reinvestment Act, which included significant health care funding, including $87 billion in additional federal matching funds for Medicaid, $25 billion for COBRA subsidies, and more than $30 billion in other health-related spending.[3]

February 26, 2009   The FY2010 budget proposal includes a more than $630 billion reserve fund to cover part of the cost of health care reform.[4]

March 5, 2009   The White House holds a forum on health care reform that includes a wide array of Administration officials; prominent members of Congress; and representatives for insurance companies, patients, doctors, hospitals, and the pharmaceutical industry.

Battles over House and Senate Legislation

May 11, 2009   Six major advocates in the health care industry—the Advanced Medical Technology Association (AdvaMed), the American Hospital Association (AHA), Pharmaceutical Researchers and Manufacturers of America (PhRMA), the American Medical Association (AMA), America's Health Insurance Plans (AHIP), and Service Employees International Union (SEIU)—sign onto a letter nominally supporting reform of health care and offering some voluntary cost-cutting measures.

June 15, 2009   President Obama addresses the AMA, saying "one essential step on our journey is to control the spiraling cost of health care in America. And in order to do that, we're going to need the help of the AMA."

July 14, 2009   Three House committees—Energy and Commerce, Ways and Means, and Education and Labor—all agree on a single health care bill, the House Tri-Committee America's Affordable Health Choices Act (H.B. 3200).

July 15, 2009   The Senate Health, Education, Labor, and Pensions (HELP) Committee passes their version of health care reform legislation, the Affordable Health Choices Act (S. 1679).

August 2009	During the August recess, members of Congress confront angry constituents at town halls. Senator Grassley (R-IA), who had been a key negotiator in an effort to produce bipartisan health care reform, argues for a much narrower bill.[5]
August 16, 2009	The President signals his willingness to drop the public option.[6]
September 9, 2009	President Obama addresses a joint session of Congress urging action on health care reform. He reiterates his priorities for this legislation, including an end to pre-existing conditions and a new insurance exchange. He does not insist upon the inclusion of a public option, and emphasizes the need for deficit reduction.
October 13, 2009	The Senate Finance Committee approves their version of health care reform, the America's Health Future Act, by a vote of 14 to 9.
November 7, 2009	By a vote of 220 to 215, the House passes health care legislation, the Affordable Health Care for America Act, H.R. 3962. The final bill includes the "Stupak Amendment," which restricts abortion coverage.
December 12, 2009	Senator Lieberman's unexpected opposition to the Senate bill leads Senator Reid to remove a buy-in to Medicare for those 55+ and the opt-out public option that had previously been included in the legislation.
December 24, 2009	The Senate passes their health care bill, the Patient Protection and Affordable Care Act, H.R. 3590.
January 15, 2010	The President and top House and Senate Democrats agree on revisions to legislation, including—after extensive consultation with union officials—a tax on high-cost insurance plans.

Scott Brown Election and the Legislative Endgame

January 19, 2010   Republican Scott Brown defeats Democrat Martha Coakley to fill the Senate seat long held by Senator Edward Kennedy. Though the White House's preferred strategy is to pass the Senate bill in the House,[7] Speaker Nancy Pelosi argues that she cannot get the votes in the House to pass an un-amended Senate version of the bill.[8] A two-step strategy, with House passage of the Senate bill followed by a bill of revisions passed under reconciliation, is rumored.[9]

January 27, 2010   President Obama delivers a State of the Union that renews the call for health care reform and warns Democrats dispirited by the Brown upset that "we still have the largest majority in decades and the people expect us to solve some problems, not run for the hills."

February 2010   Massive rate increases by Anthem Blue Cross spark national outrage.

February 22, 2010   For the first time, President Obama releases a specific policy proposal for health care reform. His recommendation closely mirrors the Senate legislation.

February 25, 2010   President Obama leads the Bipartisan Meeting on Health Care Reform. Interviewed on CNN, White House Senior Advisor David Axelrod pushes an "up or down vote" on health care reform.

March 3, 2010   President Obama gives a speech calling for action on health care reform. "I, therefore, ask leaders in both houses of Congress to finish their work and schedule a vote in the next few weeks. From now until then, I will do everything in my power to make the case for reform."

March 20, 2010	As Pelosi nears the necessary vote total to pass the Senate bill, President Obama rallies the House Democratic Caucus.
March 21, 2010	By a vote of 219 to 212, the House of Representatives passes the Senate version of health care reform, the Patient Protection and Affordable Care Act, H.R. 3590. By a vote of 220 to 211, the House passes the "sidecar" bill that revises the Senate legislation, the Health Care and Education Reconciliation Act, H.R. 4872.
March 23, 2010	President Obama signs the first part of the health care legislation, the Patient Protection and Affordable Care Act, into law. Attorneys general in fourteen states sue to block healthcare reform law.
March 26, 2010	After numerous delays, the Senate votes for the reconciliation fixes, the Health Care and Education Reconciliation Act, by a vote of 56 to 43. Procedural questions raised by Senate Republicans force the House to vote on the legislation again. It passes a second time, 220 to 207.
March 30, 2010	President Obama signs Health Care and Education Reconciliation Act into law.
October 2010– February 2011	Five separate constitutional challenges, supported by 26 states, are argued in District Courts around the country.
November 2010	In sweeping wins, Republicans gain 6 seats in the U.S. Senate, 64 seats in the U.S. House, 6 state governorships, and control of 15 state houses and 7 state senates.
January 2011 to Fall 2012	The Republican-led House passes more than 30 bills or amendments that call for repeal of the Affordable Care Act, but all such efforts are defeated or buried in the Democratic Senate.

June 2011– November 2011	Four of five Appeals Courts—the last battle lines before the Supreme Court—left the Affordable Care Act standing and decided against those claiming it was unconstitutional.
June 28, 2012	A five to four majority of the Supreme Court upholds most of the Affordable Care Act as constitutional and rules that states may refuse the proffered funds for Medicaid expansions.

1

WHY NOW? BROKEN HEALTH CARE AND AN OPPORTUNITY FOR CHANGE

Major reforms such as Social Security, Civil Rights, or Medicare are enacted in American democracy only when the stars align just right. Problems such as elderly poverty or racial oppression can fester for a very long time before reforms are even attempted—and attempts can fall short and backfire on leaders who try to address intractable dilemmas.

So it was with health reform in the late-twentieth-century United States. Gaps in health insurance coverage and rapidly rising costs for families and businesses were long-standing as well as accelerating problems. Yet many leaders in both major political parties came to political grief in failed attempts to address these difficulties. The most recent failure, spectacular and politically costly to its sponsor, was President Bill Clinton's abortive push for universal health security in 1993 and 1994. The aftermath brought a conservative Republican takeover of Congress in November 1994.[1]

To see why yet another big push for comprehensive health reform emerged in 2009, we need to understand how the 2008 election opened the door. Even more pointedly, we must explore why an unanticipated, steep economic downturn ended up reinforcing rather than deflecting the determination of newly installed President Barack Obama to move ahead on health reform. Economic anxieties and dwindling tax revenues would make health reform even more politically risky, but

Obama chose to use his agenda-setting authority to call for comprehensive reform. The growing problems in U.S. health care could not wait. The moment of possibility presented by the first year after a presidential election for change could not be missed.

WHY DOES THE COUNTRY NEED CHANGES IN HEALTH CARE?

"So You Think You're Insured? (Think Again)" was the attention-grabbing headline on the cover of the March 16, 2009, issue of *Time* magazine, which hit newsstands shortly after President Obama convened a White House summit on health care reform, declaring that he was determined to address "one of the greatest threats, not just to the well-being of our families and the prosperity of our businesses, but to the very foundation of our economy . . . the exploding cost of health care in America today."[2] The *Time* cover story by Karen Tumulty, one of the country's most knowledgeable and respected health care reporters, told the riveting story of what happened when serious illness suddenly struck her brother Pat, an "administrative assistant for a lighting firm in San Antonio."[3]

It had been six years since Pat Tumulty held a job that included health insurance coverage. While working at other jobs and looking for another position with health benefits, he had been "faithfully paying premiums to Assurant Health, buying a series of six-month medical policies" that the company's Web site told him would protect against "unexpected" illnesses and accidents that "happen every day," leading to medical bills that "can be disastrous."[4] "Safeguard your financial future with Short Term Medical temporary insurance," the Assurant Web site said. "It provides the peace of mind and health care access you need at a price you can afford." Pat's stopgap policies from Assurant had to be renewed every six months and had such a high deductible—requiring him to pay for basic health care services from his modest wages—that Pat put off going to the doctor until he was really ill. Alas, when tests confirmed that Patrick was suffering from kidney failure, Assurant found a loophole that allowed them to designate his costly illness a "preexisting condition" so the company could refuse to pay his quickly mounting bills. Pat Tumulty's insurance proved worthless just when he really needed it.

What is more, hospitals were charging Pat their highest rates for tests and procedures, because he was not covered by either a large group-health-insurance plan or a government plan that can bargain for the lowest prices. Although he is a regular taxpayer, public programs were not an obvious source of help, either, because Pat lives in Texas. Texas is a state with one of the weakest safety nets, among the least generous public programs to help the uninsured, in which only the very poor, whose income is only 26% of poverty, qualify, and then only adults with children. Not surprisingly, the uninsured constitute about a quarter of the state's population.[5]

Fortunately, Pat has an expert, well-connected sister who eventually found a county program that could help with future expenses, even as she pressured Assurant to "make an exception" and cover some of his early bills. (Would Assurant have done this for someone whose sister was not a national health reporter?) Pat's health and financial situation remained tenuous as Karen wrote her cover story in early 2009, using her family's experience with the big gaps left by America's patchwork of private and public health insurance programs to make a larger point: "What makes…cases" like Patrick's "terrifying in addition to heartbreaking, is that they reveal the hard truth about this country's health-care system: just about anyone could be one bad diagnosis away from financial ruin."[6]

Shrinking Access to Affordable Care

Tumulty's point is obvious for close to 38 million working-aged Americans and family members who do not enjoy insurance coverage.[7] Almost three-quarters of these unfortunate uninsured people work, more than half of them full-time.[8] For decades, the uninsured in America have typically been not the rich or the very poor, but members of families whose bread-winner (or breadwinners) were employed at low or modest wages, usually in small businesses.[9] Tellingly, inequalities in employee access to health insurance have become steadily worse—and the situation for low-paid workers is scandalously bad.[10] From around 1980 to the present, relatively privileged employees in the top two-fifths of the wage scale have experi-enced some erosion in health coverage, but more than 90% of such high earners continue to enjoy insurance. Employees in the middle fifth of the wage distribution have gone from around 5% uninsured to 12.4% without health coverage, a worrisome trend to be sure, but nothing compared to the loss of coverage by those below them in the wage scale. Lower-middle-wage earners in the next-to-bottom fifth have gone from less than 10% uninsured to 21.9% without health insur-ance, and low-wage earners in the bottom fifth have gone from 18% to a whopping 37.4% lacking health coverage. These are U.S. citizens who work as janitors or clerks or health care assis-tants day after day, week after week, year after year, contrib-uting to our economy and doing right by their families and communities.

But even people who appear to be covered by employer or individual insurance policies can be in for an abrupt surprise if serious illness strikes, because another 16 million are underin-sured or lack coverage for catastrophic medical expenses.[11] Perhaps their employers' plans have fine print limiting total payouts to far less than what it takes to treat a catastrophic ill-ness; or perhaps their small business employers can no longer afford coverage if rates are suddenly hiked after one employee falls ill. Or, perhaps, as happened to Patrick Tumulty, an indi-vidually purchased policy is canceled when the insurers root out some retrospective hint that the person might have been getting sick before he or she purchased the policy. The person does not even have to know a bad diagnosis is on the way, to suffer a rescission of coverage after the fact. A report by *Reuters* news agency revealed that "tens of thousands of Americans lost their health insurance shortly after being diagnosed with life-threatening, expensive medical conditions," and cited findings by Congress that the insurance giant, WellPoint, has been a "worst offender," because the company routinely scoured the records of female policyholders newly diagnosed with breast cancer, trying to find some hint of a "pre-existing" illness of any sort that would allow cancellation of the policies before the company had to pay high treatment costs.[12]

Paying More for Less

Huge and growing gaps in insurance coverage might make some sense if the United States were especially frugal about health care compared to other advanced nations. Maybe the United States just wants to save money. But the opposite is true. The United States spends about twice as much per person as other industrial countries do on average, and more than 50% more than the next-biggest spender, eating up a huge and growing chunk of what our national economy produces.[13] According to the Organization for Economic Co-Operation and Development (OECD), which tracks trends in 31 industrialized nations, U.S. health spending in 2006 amounted to 15.3% of Gross Domestic Product (GDP, a measure of a country's total economic output), and that was far higher than the other 30 economically affluent democracies.[14] Our neighbor to the north, Canada, spent 10% of GDP; France spent 11%, Germany 10.6%, and Britain 8.4%; and the second-biggest spender, Switzerland, devoted 11.3% of GDP to health care. What is more, heath care costs in the United States have also escalated at a much higher rate than those of sister nations. Since the 1970s, America's health care costs have risen at a rate over 2 percentage points faster than GDP, which explains why the chunk of national productivity devoted to health care expanded sharply—from about 7.2% of GDP in 1970, to 15.3% in 2006 (and a projected 17.6% in 2009).[15]

America's outsized spending on health care is particularly worrisome given that all other industrial nations *provide their entire populations with health coverage.* They do it in a lot of different ways, sometimes with a central role for government, but in some instances like Germany and Switzerland by regulating private insurance companies and helping all citizens afford coverage. However they manage to ensure universal health care, other nations get hugely more bang for the buck than the United States does, and they manage to keep a tighter rein on rising health-care costs.[16]

Defenders of the status quo in U.S. health care often argue back against such unflattering international comparisons. America has the most technologically advanced health care in the world, the finest hospitals and most expert doctors, they declare. And defenders of the current system point out that, really, all Americans have access to medical care, because anyone can get help by turning up at a hospital emergency room.

Advanced technology, however, can raise costs if it is used wastefully—as it often is in the United States when well-insured patients are at issue and doctors or hospitals have an incentive to provide costly tests or treatments. If your income or profit margins depend on doing a lot of MRIs or running that extra test, why not do it for well-insured patients—especially if you want to make sure you are not accused of malpractice?[17] Despite extra tests and procedures and defensive medicine, though, international measures of health care results show that American patients in general often do worse than people with comparable conditions in other, more frugal national health care systems.[18] Our infant-mortality rate ranks twenty-eighth among the nations of the world, and we have much more marked differences in health outcomes by race and ethnicity than other major nations. Sister industrial nations do better at helping people survive childhood leukemia and various adult cancers, and access to immediate care is often more difficult for Americans than for citizens of comparable nations, such as Canada and Britain. America may do the very best for its most privileged people, those with the best insurance coverage who have lots of inside connections and are savvy about how to navigate the system. But, overall, we cannot justify our broken-down patchwork system by saying it delivers better health results.

As for that emergency room argument: certainly, if you manage to stagger in, some hospital will patch up "a bullet hole in...[the] chest"—as the chief of staff to conservative Republican senatorial candidate Sue Lowden of Arizona put it in a May 2010 interview, trying to make the case that every American has access to health care.[19] Indeed, a recent study documents that an estimated one-fifth of 120 million hospital emergency room visits in 2006 were by uninsured people.[20] But emergency rooms cannot provide routine preventive care or deal with ongoing conditions. As their name says, emergency rooms are supposed to be available for sudden crises that can happen to anyone, such as a severe injury in a car accident. If emergency rooms are clogged with uninsured people looking for many kinds of help, they cannot do their vital primary job for all of us—after all, any one of us or a loved one could be turned away by an overcrowded emergency room, diverted to a different hospital when minutes could count to save life or limb. Faced with mounting costs, many private hospitals are closing emergency rooms; and public hospitals that, by law, must take all comers are struggling at a time of cutbacks in taxpayer subsidies.[21]

The truth is that emergency care as a substitute for affordable normal access is often neither appropriate nor cost-effective; and of course it is not truly "free." Hospital bill collectors may hound nonpaying patients for years thereafter, and if the bills cannot be collected, costs are shifted onto everyone else. Hospitals charge paying patients higher rates; governments raise taxes to subsidize public and teaching hospitals; physicians have to forgive fees to help needy patients without insurance; and insurance companies jack up premiums for everyone.[22] In short, all of us pay for care awkwardly and sporadically delivered to uninsured people, who often wait until health problems are really bad before presenting themselves at the emergency room.

HOW DID IT COME TO THIS?

Given Americans' can-do spirit, how did our country's health care system get to this sorry impasse? Thousands of books and articles, entire libraries, have traced the history of U.S. health care and insurance coverage, and we cannot present all the findings and arguments here. But it is not hard to encapsulate the basic story of how the United States created its paradoxical approach to health care—featuring high costs, patchwork, and unequal coverage, and lots of innovation along with uneven quality in health outcomes.

Between the late 1800s and the end of World War II (Bismarck pushed through health insurance in the 1880s), most other advanced industrial nations created systems of universal health insurance coverage, and reform proponents in the United States tried to find ways to do the same here.[23] Reform efforts repeatedly fell short, and private health insurance developed as an alternative, under the watchful eye of doctors who were wary (with reason as it turned out) that they and their patients would come under the tutelage of the insurance industry.

The failure to enact national health insurance culminated in an especially consequential failure at a key turning point, just after World War II, when President Harry Truman's call for universal health insurance was rejected by Congress. This happened around the same time that Congress encouraged widespread hospital building and the federal government and private foundations sharply increased funding for innovative health-related research, even as U.S. pharmaceutical giants devised a steady stream of new drugs that would be extraordinarily profitable and protected by

U.S. patents. After World War II, in short, the U.S. government encouraged innovative, profitable health care but left many citizens out of health coverage.[24] From then on, established special interests and more privileged categories of citizens would not need to ally with the remaining uninsured; the "haves" in health care could get more without the "have nots" being included.

From 1946 through the 1960s, it looked as if things might work out anyway.[25] Even in the absence of governmentally assured universal health insurance, growing proportions of middle-class Americans gained access to effective health care. Trade unions were newly enlarged and empowered after the New Deal, and they bargained with industrial giants like General Motors and U.S. Steel for generous employer-arranged health benefits. Regardless of union contracts, most larger U.S. businesses expanded their offerings of privately purchased and tax-subsidized health insurance to cover both waged workers and white-collar employees and executives. After all, employers could get generous tax breaks for such benefits, and in the early postwar period they were offering insurance to a relatively youthful workforce. (Large numbers of insured retirees would bring much higher costs later, but that was down the road.)

Health insurance reformers after World War II concentrated on pushing for what became, in 1965, the federal Medicare insurance program covering much of the expense of physician and hospital care for the retired elderly, plus the federal-state Medicaid program, covering some of the very poor, especially nonworking mothers and their children.[26] Reformers aimed to establish public responsibility first for categories of people not attractive to private insurers, and then hope that remaining uninsured Americans would either be absorbed by expanding public-health insurance programs or covered by expansions in tax-subsidized employer-provided insurance.

As late as the 1970s, it looked like this bifurcated approach to a distinctively U.S. system of health care coverage might succeed in doing in a different way what other advanced nations achieved with their various sorts of universal insurance systems. But then the cost of health care rapidly rose, due to the unrestrained use of technology and the chaotic and perverse financial incentives of America's unique approach to medical reimbursement.[27]

As Medicare payments to doctors and hospitals bloated the budget deficit, President Ronald Reagan suspended his small government ideology in deference to his fiscal conservatism and initiated direct government control over the program's spending—a step that Presidents John Kennedy and Lyndon Johnson had resisted two decades earlier out of fear of big-government criticism from Reagan and other critics of Medicare.[28] Even as Medicare started to use its bargaining power to keep price increases under control, private health care expenditures rapidly grew. Employer-provided benefits, along with policies purchased by individuals on the private insurance market, saw their premiums increase at rates faster than growth in business profits or wages. Small businesses not able to bargain with private insurers on behalf of huge pools of patients faced the highest prices and greatest risks of sudden increases; many small businesses never offered coverage and others had to cut back. Larger employers faced with steadily mounting premiums shifted more and more of the cost onto their workers, either directly by charging higher employee contributions or indirectly by holding back wage increases to defray health costs. And, of course, the work opportunities and work lives of many Americans changed in the late twentieth century. In recent times, more and more employees are classified as part-time workers, "temps," or independent contractors—allowing businesses to arrange for their services without paying fully (if at all) toward health or retirement benefits. Self-employed men and women must pay very high premiums on the small-group or individual health insurance market if they are to obtain coverage at all.

From the late 1970s, it became apparent that the fill-in-the-gaps approach to including almost all Americans with basic health insurance was faltering. Each successive year, about a million additional working-age people found themselves without health coverage—even though public programs like Medicaid or the State Children's Insurance Program expanded from time to time to cover some additional needy people. Subtly but perceptibly the concerns of businesses, employees, families, and governments shifted toward controlling rising prices and costs, not covering more people.

Around the time that President Bill Clinton tried and failed to pass his Health Security plan in the early 1990s, privately brokered experiments in managed care created some cost savings and moderated rising prices for health insurance for a few years, even as robust economic growth and expansions of public programs allowed the proportion of the population covered by insurance to hold steady for a bit in the late 1990s.[29] But with the arrival of unified Republican governance in Washington, DC, during the two presidential terms of George Bush Jr., from 2000 through 2007, public programs for the poor stalled, and sluggish economic growth hurt employers and workers. Health insurance premiums resumed their upward trajectory, and many employers either dropped coverage or required employees to contribute more to the cost. The one key extension of health benefits under Bush was the addition of a prescription drug benefit to Medicare—helpful to millions of seniors, though not paid for by new revenues, which meant that Medicare was projected to increase federal deficits still more rapidly in coming decades.

In the years just before 2008, rising costs meant that increasing numbers of people, with coverage through jobs or individually purchased plans, paid more for less adequate insurance. Many insured people face higher deductibles (meaning they have to pay the first several thousand in health care costs each year) or have to pay fees each time they visit the doctor (even $10 to $15 per visit can add up fast for patients in need of ongoing care). Scholars have also recorded sharp increases in the numbers of nominally insured people who do not have adequate coverage to protect them against high out-of-pocket expenses in an emergency—with *high* defined as costs totally more than 10% of family income. Whether insured or not, families struggling with high out-of-pocket expenses are, as a key study puts it, "more likely than other families to report difficulties in obtaining needed care, and often have trouble paying their bills—increasing the possibility that they may face debt or bankruptcy."[30] Indeed, catastrophic health care costs are a leading cause of family bankruptcy in today's America.[31]

Meanwhile, employers have been reaching the breaking point with escalating health premiums. As Figure 1.1 vividly dramatizes, from 1999 to the start of the Obama reform debate in 2009, employers offering family health coverage to their employees had to cover a remarkable 131% increase in premiums—and they did so in large part by shifting much of the cost to the contributions their employees have to make to health coverage. These covered employees were, in effect, the lucky ones in our country, because at least they enjoyed access to health insurance purchased at a rate negotiated for larger pools of people. But even these relatively fortunate insured Americans were paying sharply more for coverage, especially over the course of the first decade of the twenty-first century. Insured employees in America today face their own versions of escalating health costs and fears about how to pay, just like fellow citizens who are self-employed, or those working as temps, part-timers, or independent contractors, as well as the uninsured trying to get by without any safety net. Given the astronomical growth in health care costs, many Americans are preoccupied with affording higher fees or contributions, not to mention covering extra health care costs that might pop up with serious or chronic illnesses. Even the elderly on Medicare can have that worry, because prescription drugs could be very pricey for millions of them who fell into the "doughnut hole" gap left in the federal plan—a hole that meant especially high out-of-pocket costs for people with chronic conditions requiring drugs costing more than a couple of thousand dollars a year.[32]

To summarize our whirlwind overview: For more than sixty years, our democracy has encouraged—and subsidized—profit-making businesses, researchers, and medical professionals, unleashing them to create wondrous medical innovations and make money by offering advanced health care—and by selling insurance for fortunate segments of the population, especially privileged employees and their families. But many in the working and middle class are falling into growing cracks, as more and more employers and families are being priced out of secure access to health care. No wonder that seven or eight out of every ten Americans have been consistently insisting that the health system needed fundamental change or needed to be completely rebuilt.[33] The riches of health care beckon to frustrated and fearful people who need it, but it is as if growing portions of the American citizenry find themselves on rafts close to idyllic shores yet pulled outward by currents against

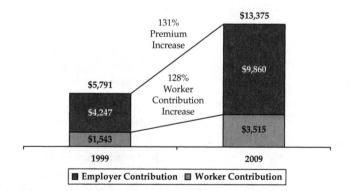

Figure 1.1. Average Health Insurance Premiums and Worker Contributions for Family Coverage, 1999–2009. *Note*: The average worker contribution and the average employer contribution may not add to the average total premium due to rounding. *Source*: Kaiser/HRET Survey of Employer-Sponsored Health Benefits, 1999–2000.

which their oars, no matter how vigorously rowed, can make only limited headway.

This was already the situation as of 2007 and 2008, as U.S. voters looked toward the next presidential election, where they could express hopes and anxieties that had built for some time. Along with the sluggish economy, affordable health care was one of people's top concerns as the election cycle started.

HOW AN ELECTION FOR CHANGE PAVED THE WAY FOR (ANOTHER ATTEMPT AT) HEALTH REFORM

The 2008 election opened the door to comprehensive health care reform because it led to convincing Democratic victories in Congress as well as the presidency. But puzzles remain: Barack Obama was *not* the Democrat most identified with health care reform during the primary election. How did he deepen his commitment to comprehensive health reform in debates with other Democrats, and then highlight health care issues in the general election competition with John McCain?

Health Care in the Democratic Primaries

As the 2008 presidential election campaign started back in 2007, Americans were disillusioned with outgoing Republican President George W. Bush and Republicans in Congress, who had promoted the protracted war in Iraq, bungled the Hurricane Katrina disaster, and refused to move on even incremental reforms amidst a sluggish and then deteriorating economy. Republicans had, for example, never put forward any proposals for national health reform during years in unified control of the Presidency and both houses of Congress. What is more, after the 2006 election resulted in massive gains for Democrats in Congress, President Bush had repeatedly vetoed bipartisan legislation to extend coverage to more children in the State Children's Health Insurance Program, denying low-wage families one of the few fallbacks they could use during a period of eroding coverage from hard-pressed employers.

As Democrats geared up during 2007 for their party's primaries, they were optimistic that their party would have a very good chance to take the presidency and make additional headway in Congress. Comprehensive health care reform was a longstanding party priority—intensely popular with rank and file Democrats and with many Independents who vote in Democratic primaries. For the first time in a decade and a half, the fearfulness to take up reform that hung around after the Clinton failure in 1994, was dissipating. Plans were regularly discussed to extend coverage to the uninsured, regulate insurance company practices—and, many Democrats hoped, to create a "public option" to let working-age Americans buy public coverage like Medicare.

By general consensus, the early frontrunner for the Democratic nomination was New York Senator and former First Lady Hillary Rodham Clinton—deemed a formidable candidate to beat throughout the summer and fall of 2007.[34] Former North Carolina Senator John Edwards also looked as if he had a good shot, because he had run strongly in the Iowa Caucuses in 2004 and the Iowa contest would be the first to be held, on January 3, 2008, kicking off the official Democratic primary season. Meanwhile, the junior Senator from Illinois, Barack Obama, aroused considerable interest from major Democratic donors and from many young people after he declared for the presidency on February 10, 2007, in Springfield, Illinois. All three of these frontrunners claimed a commitment to doing major health care reforms, but Clinton and Edwards were bolder and more specific in the early going.

Tellingly, health care was featured at the very first Democratic presidential forum focused on specific issues. Held on March 24, 2007, at the University of Las Vegas, the forum was co-sponsored by the Service Employees Union—a major player in the party's electoral base—and the Center for American Progress (CAP)—an influential DC think tank preparing governing agendas for the next Democratic president. As moderator, Karen Tumulty posed specific and well-informed questions to the Democratic contenders. John Edwards made it clear that he had commissioned experts to draw up a detailed plan for universal coverage and cost controls. Hillary Rodham Clinton was in her element, showing an unparalleled depth of knowledge as she explained what she had learned from the failed Clinton effort of 1993–1994. "She was sharp, passionate, and detailed; the crowd ate it up," in the words of journalists John Heilemann and Mark Halperin.[35] Obama, by contrast, was "only casually prepared" and assumed "he could wing it." "Vague and platitudinous, mouthing generalities and making excuses for not having his health plan in order, Obama came across as amateurish. The union audience was both surprised and mildly offended."[36] Still, Obama did make a clear promise, saying "I will judge my first term as president based on... whether we have delivered the kind of health care that every American deserves and that our system can afford."[37]

This may have been bold, but as Democratic presidential contenders spelled out their health reform plans throughout the interminable primary season, Obama offered ideas that seemed cautious and short of a commitment to try for universal coverage. True, Obama's image as a progressive Democratic primary candidate rested in part on his race and his fresh appeal to young voters, and in even larger part on his much-touted early public opposition to the War in Iraq: Obama gave a speech opposing George Bush's war back in 2002, while both Senator Clinton and Senator Edwards had voted that fall to authorize Bush to proceed toward what became the invasion of Iraq. The Democratic primary electorate held those votes against Clinton and Edwards—and especially against Clinton, because, unlike Edwards, she refused simply to apologize for her vote. But the fact was that on health care, one of the leading domestic issues for Democratic activists, unionists, and primary voters, the supposedly progressive Obama was not only slow to spell out his plan (it finally appeared in October 2007) but also promised less than Edwards and Clinton on a key issue: whether he would eventually require every American to purchase health coverage, once public subsidies were in place. As the protracted Democratic battles moved from Iowa, where Obama won resoundingly, aided by antiwar voters and young first-time caucus goers, to such hardscrabble places as Ohio and Pennsylvania, Clinton was well positioned to hammer Obama with female, working-class, and older voters. She would make sure the country reached universal health coverage, she claimed, by helping everyone to pay for coverage and requiring everyone to join the system. She spoke caustically of Obama's unwillingness to guarantee anything more than full coverage for children. "Senator Obama's plan does not, and cannot, cover all Americans. He called his plan universal, then he called it "virtually universal," but it is not either," Senator Clinton argued in a November 2007 speech in Iowa, "When it comes to truth in labeling, it simply flunks the test."[38]

Ultimately, of course, Obama accumulated the most delegates across all the Democratic primary states, winning major victories in a number of mass primaries—such as South Carolina, Maryland, and Wisconsin—and also securing delegates in sixteen caucus states, where the delegate count was determined by activists turning out at meetings. Hillary Rodham Clinton, however, remained in contention until the very end of the fifty-six primaries and caucuses. Arguably, by competing so long with Clinton, Obama learned to address lunch-bucket Democrats on economic issues, including working women who were especially concerned with access and cost in health care. Certainly, he visibly gained more passion and specificity on these issues by the late spring of 2008. Nevertheless, Obama always remained more cautious than Clinton on politically tricky specifics—like the "individual mandate," which his advisors feared might be used against him in the general election campaign, if Republicans could claim he wanted to coerce or tax Americans. In the primaries, Obama hammered on "affordability" as the key health-care issue. Virtually all Americans, he claimed, would voluntarily buy health coverage if it were made affordable with price cuts and subsidies. Again and again, Clinton reported that reform could not be effective unless everyone, not just children, were included in truly universal health coverage.

Obama Makes Health Care His Issue

The primaries dragged on until the last two states, Montana and South Dakota, voted on June 3, 2008. Obama only sealed the Democratic nomination with the support of "superdelegates," party leaders not elected through the nomination contest. After Clinton's concession speech on Saturday, June 7, he moved quickly to reach out to her millions of primary supporters. Obama desperately needed Clinton's voters in the looming general election contest with John McCain, including the enthusiastic support of independent and Democratic women disappointed at the lost chance to nominate a female for president. Knowing that health care was an issue where he could repeatedly praise Hillary and touch the hearts of women, Obama subtly shifted toward his erstwhile rival—certainly in his rhetoric and display of passion for universal health care. As he pulled a number of Clinton's political and policy advisors into his organization, Obama recruited Neera Tanden, an expert on health care who had run Clinton's policy operation. From the start of the general election campaign, Obama touted his commitment "to make health care affordable for every single American" while declaring that Republican presumptive nominee John McCain "like George Bush,...has a plan that takes care only of the healthy and wealthy."[39]

Obama laid down his marker at one of his very first events after clinching the Democratic nomination, at a Health Care Town Hall Meeting, held in Bristol, Virginia, on June 5, 2008, where he addressed the crowd using health-care stories about individual Americans to blend his longstanding stress on the poll-tested theme of affordability with the goal of health care coverage for all, which he knew to be music to the ears of Democrats, especially erstwhile Clinton supporters. "You know," Obama said,

> I've been traveling across America on this campaign for 16 months now, and everywhere I've gone, I've heard heartbreaking stories about our health care system.
>
> There's the young woman I met who works the night shift after a full day of college and still can't afford medicine for a sister who's ill; or the man I met who almost lost his home because he has three children with cystic fibrosis and couldn't pay their health care bills; who still doesn't have health insurance for himself or his wife and lives in fear that a single illness could cost them everything....
>
> I don't think the American people can afford another four years of a health care plan that does more to help the big drug and insurance companies than it does to lower costs for ordinary Americans. We need to make health care affordable for every single American, and that's what I'll do as president.[40]

Obama's presidential campaign returned again and again to the promise of affordable health care for all Americans. It was one of his themes as he accepted the Democratic nomination in a dramatic mass rally that included Obama volunteers as well as Convention delegates, held under starry skies at Mile High Stadium in Denver on the night of Thursday, August 28, 2008. "America, now is not the time for small plans," Obama declared, as he derided McCain for wanting to continue "failed" policies of President Bush and the Republicans and called for bold actions to renew a "threatened" American promise. Among the actions, Obama pledged, would be comprehensive health care reform, with the goals of his plan specified in more detail than other policies mentioned in the address. "Now is the time to finally keep the promise of affordable, accessible health care for every single American," Obama said. "If you have health care, my plan will lower your premiums. If you don't, you'll be able to get the same kind of coverage that members of Congress give themselves."[41] In September and October, Obama continued to feature health care reform in debates and campaign ads, even as the Wall Street meltdown and deepening national economic downturn overtook the campaigns of both contending candidates in the final weeks before November 5.

Still, it is worth emphasizing that Obama's campaign against John McCain remained politically cautious where potentially controversial aspects of health care reform were at issue. Obama took stands in the heat of the election that he would change as President, when he had to make decisions with an eye to costs and workability. For instance, during the election itself, Obama never did clearly commit to the notion of an "individual mandate" that would require all Americans, in due course, to have insurance; and on a matter close to the hearts of progressives in his own party, Obama danced around the "public option," repeatedly, praising the notion that Americans should be able to choose between private and public insurance options, but without drawing any "line in the sand" about what eventual reform legislation would have to include.

Above all, Obama was wary during the general election about anything that could be called a health care tax on the middle class. Many experts want to control rising health insurance costs in the future in part by rolling back the longstanding federal tax breaks that allow employers to offer especially generous health plans to employees. Generous tax-advantaged employer plans, eventually dubbed "Cadillac plans," are provided to executives, managers, and professional employees of big businesses and non-profit organizations (such as Harvard University, where one of the authors of this book works). In addition, over the decades since health insurance became part of collective bargaining in the 1940s, many unions like the United Mine Workers have bargained for good health coverage for their members and retirees. Naturally, businesses that provide tax-advantaged health plans, along with employees and union members who enjoy especially capacious coverage, do not want to see the price of their insurance go up in the future because it is taxed, even if adjustments in the federal tax code would help to control health premium increases across the system as a whole. During the 2008 general election, Obama remained sensitive to business and union opposition to trimming the tax advantages enjoyed by Cadillac plans. Indeed, the Obama campaign criticized John McCain's health reform plan for proposing to abolish the special tax advantages of employer-provided health insurance. And as the presidential contest reached a crescendo in October 2008, the Obama campaign released a hard-hitting television commercial attacking McCain's health proposals as a new plan, "taxing health benefits for the first time ever," and concluding "we can't afford John McCain."[42] Ironically, once he became President, Obama would eventually accept a version of a future tax on Cadillac plans. But in the campaign itself, he tailored his health reform themes for popular understanding and electoral advantage, just as he had done in response to Hillary Rodham Clinton during earlier phases of the presidential marathon.

Obama's cautious tailoring of his message to deflect Republican charges reflected a more durable reality about American culture that would guide how Democrats designed reform after the election. Although more than 70% of Americans were dissatisfied with the health system's cost and insurance coverage, they were quite satisfied with the quality of their personal care and leery of disruptive government changes; a series of Gallup polls after 2001 found steady majorities in favor of maintaining private health insurance instead of a "new government-run health care system."[43] This public ambivalence led Obama to campaign on broad homilies about affordability and cost, and after the election the reality of public ambivalence would hover over his efforts to deliver "change" without unnerving Americans.

A NEW PRESIDENT WITH AN AGENDA FOR CHANGE

As everyone knows, the 2008 presidential election finally resulted in a resounding victory for Barack Obama, who beat McCain by 53% to 46% in the popular vote, and carried 28 states with 365 Electoral College votes versus 22 states with 173 Electoral College votes for McCain. So badly beaten were the Republicans in the contests for Congress as well as in the presidential contest that respected commentators speculated that the new President was ideally positioned to carry through a "New New Deal"—to cite the cover story on the November 24, 2008, issue of *Time*, which pictured a jaunty-looking Obama riding like FDR in an open convertible with a long holder for his cigarette jutting from his smiling lips. Some analysts also suggested that Democrats could be on the verge of accomplishing a permanent electoral "realignment," because they had ridden surges in voter participation in 2006 through 2008, and their supporters included growing demographics within the national electorate: African Americans and Latinos, young people, college-educated people, and working women.[44]

To be sure, others remained dubious, noting that Americans are inherently cautious about government initiatives, and the recession would probably leave too many millions jobless for too long. The next election, in the fall of 2010, could arrive well before full economic recovery, especially in the job market; the voters who usually turn out in mid-term elections are whiter and older and richer people, exactly the demographics least approving of Obama. But for months such worries seemed misplaced, as Americans reported optimism that the popular new President would soon turn the economy around.[45]

Obama lined up most officials for his Cabinet and White House teams even before the January 20 inauguration, mobbed by some two million celebrants stretching like a sea of humanity in the midst of Washington, DC. One glitch would prove worrisome for health reform: Obama planned to name former Senate Majority Leader and South Dakota Senator Tom Daschle as both his Secretary of Health and Human Services and his key White House coordinator for health policy. But in his recent years in DC, since losing his Senate seat, Daschle had worked on behalf of a major health insurance conglomerate, and had neglected to pay taxes on gifts he had received as a consultant.[46] Critics seized on that mistake and forced Daschle to withdraw. This meant that Obama would not have such a major figure coordinating health reform policy between the Congress and the White House. It also meant a three-month delay before Kathleen Sebelius was eventually confirmed to Health and Human Services, while Nancy Ann DeParle took the lead from the White House side.

Fighting Recession amidst Republican Opposition

Still, Obama's administration hit the ground running with a vigorous response to the contracting economy, proposing, right after the inauguration, a bill that became the American Recovery and Reinvestment Act (the so-called stimulus) featuring $787 billion in spending and tax cuts to stimulate the economy and put in place "down payments" on policy shifts in numerous key areas, including expansions in health insurance coverage for children and the unemployed. But there were also early signs of gathering political troubles for Obama's economic and social agendas. His recovery proposal depended almost entirely on Democrats for its enactment. House Republicans voted against it down to the last man and woman; and in the Senate, only three Republicans (Maine Senators Susan Collins and Olympia Snowe plus then-Republican Arlen Specter of Pennsylvania) could be attracted to let a watered down version of the legislation eke through their chamber. The sudden coalescence of partisan opposition chagrined the

Obama White House, which had anticipated broader support for desperately needed spending relief and Republican-style business tax cuts.[47] Although the recovery proposal passed, the ominous signal sent by the determination of Republican Congressional leaders to orchestrate blanket opposition was hard to ignore.

Frightened by the extent of their losses in 2006 and 2008, and dealing with a shrunken popular base that intensely disliked Obama, Republican leaders decided to gamble on total opposition. If they supported Obama initiatives that ended up working, would Republicans get any credit? But if they opposed recovery legislation and any subsequent big initiatives such as health care reform, maybe they could both please their core conservative base *and* position themselves to be the only alternative if voters remained unhappy in a sluggish economy through 2010 and 2012. The U.S. electoral system, after all, offers only two alternatives in most elections: Democrats or Republicans. If things are not going well in the economy or in their family fortunes, voters tend to think it is better to send a distress signal and "give the other guy a chance." Republican leaders thus knew their party could benefit if President Obama and the Democrats were unable to engineer an instant economic recovery, especially if Congress could be deadlocked to prevent potentially popular legislation from passing (at least not quickly, thus allowing negative advertising to take hold). In addition to positioning themselves to benefit from bad times during Obama's term, Republicans and their allies relied on what had become standard procedure in Washington—investing tens of millions into polling to craft deceptive talking points and ads that misled Americans, leaving them with little accurate information about legislative maneuvers in Washington, DC, and suspicious about the consequences for themselves and their families.[48]

This was the lay of the land as early as February and March of Obama's first term: partisan obstruction in Washington and alarming growth in unemployment as the economy spiraled downward. As the new President got down to work, health care reform was *not* the American public's top priority—indeed it had not even been at the top back in November, when Americans were asked about their worries and priorities as of Election Day. To be sure, 66% of Americans told exit pollsters that they were worried about being able to afford health care, and three-fifths of these worriers supported Obama over McCain. But when asked to name the most important issue that the country needed to address, led by the new President, only 9% of voters said health care (about the same percentage that designated Iraq or terrorism as the most important issue), while 63% named the economy. This was hardly surprising given that, even in November, long before the job market bottomed out in early 2009, a whopping 93% of voting Americans labeled the state of the economy "poor" or "not good"; and 85% said they were worried about the economy. The overwhelming percentage worried about the deteriorating economy was substantially higher than the 66% who said they were worried about health care.[49]

Should Health Care Be Delayed?

Predictably, interest groups and commentators not so enthusiastic about comprehensive health reform under Democratic auspices quickly proclaimed that Obama had too much on his plate and should delay health reform to fix the economy first. Inside players in Washington, DC, do not really expect newly elected Presidents to carry through things they promise voters. Presidents are expected to look at issues anew and reassess once they move inside the Beltway. The (somewhat cynical) assumption is that all that campaign rhetoric is fluff to get elected, and then, once in office, presidents should listen to powerful interests and be "realistic" about keeping promises they made to voters. In this instance, even some Democratic pundits, like Bill Galston, a Clinton Administration veteran now installed at the Brookings Institution, suggested it might be prudent to go forward with health reform in small, incremental steps.[50]

Inside the White House not long after the Inauguration, a fateful debate broke out about how to use precious months of the President's first year—including his "honeymoon period" of inflated popularity likely to last no more than six months. Should they prioritize what would surely be a tough fight for comprehensive health reform? Vice President Joe Biden argued that the Administration should concentrate on the most urgent challenges facing the country: correcting the country's worst economic crisis since the Great Depression of the 1930s and reforming the financial industry to prevent future bankruptcies and financial trickery. He was backed up by heavy hitters, including the White House's top political advisor, David Axelrod, and Obama's Chief of Staff Rahm Emanuel; and Treasury Secretary Timothy Geithner pressed to make finance reform the top legislative priority.[51] These heavyweights worried that taking on health reform and other initiatives that Obama had promised during his campaign would overload Congress, distract the Administration from addressing the primary concern of Americans with jobs and restarting the economy. Obama's presidency could be at risk if they failed to get priorities right.

Although the public face of the White House projected confidence, the watchword behind the scenes was failure. After all, presidents since Teddy Roosevelt had been seduced into pursuing health reform and failed. Emanuel focused the White House and reform allies on their daunting challenge, declaring the "goal isn't to see whether I can pass this through the executive board of [a Washington think tank like the] Brookings Institution," but to get it "through the United States Congress with people who represent constituents."[52] Emanuel knew from his years as a White House aide under Bill Clinton how maddeningly difficult it is for a president to get Congress to move on something as huge and intricate as health care reform. And his bitter experiences in the early 1990s taught Emanuel the high cost of political failure on a signature presidential priority. Droves of Democrats in Congress lost in the 1994 elections after an attempt at comprehensive health reform crashed and burned. The battle-scarred Emanuel repeatedly instructed aides, "I don't want to fail."[53]

The advice of senior White House officials to delay health reform was countered by strong pressure from congressional Democrats and campaign supporters. After the November election, Senator Ted Kennedy and the powerful chair of the Senate Finance Committee, Max Baucus, met with Obama to insist that health reform be his top domestic priority after stabilizing the financial and economic systems. Baucus also wrote Obama and publicly released a White Paper on health reform to up the ante.[54] Kennedy's losing battle with brain cancer, his lifelong campaign for health reform, and his decisive endorsement of Obama during the Democratic primaries made his appeal to move ahead "incredibly emotionally freighted," in the words of a Kennedy aide, instilling in Obama a sense that he "needed to do this for Kennedy."[55]

Warnings about overloading Congress did not impress Obama. Having seen Congress operate from the inside during his years in the Senate, Obama was convinced that the separate committees could work simultaneously on an ambitious agenda, with the leadership staggering the arrival of bills called up for a vote on the floors of the House and Senate.

Those who doubted the wisdom of proceeding with comprehensive health care reform at the outset of Obama's presidency offered convincing reasons and may well have prevailed under normal circumstances. But 2009 was extraordinary and Obama challenged the assumptions of his advisors. The economic crisis had shaken many Americans and businesses, in some ways renewing the opportunity to push for health reforms that would help people get or afford health coverage. Obama saw the risks of health reform as significant, but not enough to deter an attempt to achieve something of historic importance for regular people and the nation's future.

He was also skeptical of the idea that passing a major piece of legislation would drain his political capital. Just the opposite; Obama believed that "victories would beget victories"—winning on health reform would add momentum to moving other parts of his agenda, including reform of the financial system.

Republicans and some congressional Democrats worried that health reform would explode an already over-extended budget and add to the government's debt. But officials in the Obama Administration—especially its Office of Management and the Budget led by the influential Peter Orszag—took an opposite view, namely, that well-designed health legislation was necessary to control medical care costs in the short term and reduce them over time. Health reform that emphasized cost controls along with universal access could be understood as a vital economic and fiscal measure, which could free businesses and government budgets from excessive costs. Obama's budget gurus firmly believed that federal deficits would balloon uncontrollably until there were reforms in health care spending. Those reforms had to include better controls on cost increases in the private sector and adjustments downward in projected Medicare spending. Yet Obama's experts believed it would be impossible to control health expenditures without somehow getting everyone into basic insurance coverage, because as long as "no coverage" remains an option, insurance companies and other big players can maneuver to make money by avoiding the sick, the poor, or others likely to need more medical care (such as near-retirees, 55–65 years old). Only if everyone gets included at a basic level can big players reasonably be expected to deliver care and offer insurance in new ways, looking to save and make money with efficiencies rather than exclusions.

Obama himself was sympathetic to these arguments. He understood comprehensive health reform—marrying virtually universal access to cost controls—as an alternative to across-the-board cuts in the government entitlement programs.

Nor did the President accept the idea that health reform would be a distraction from the economy. He saw it as a prerequisite to improving the competitiveness of American business by reducing its high and rising health costs. Covering everybody and getting costs under control would encourage economic innovation and growth and help to create new jobs.

Marry the fear of future deficits with Obama's realization, honed in the long election campaigns, that his Democratic Party base was expecting bold reforms to cover millions in need of affordable care, and it becomes understandable why Obama decided not to let an unexpected economic crisis divert him from the vision he laid out during his campaign. The new President wanted to lead in refashioning the foundations of the U.S. economy and social contract, laying the basis for long-term economic growth that would enlarge security and opportunity for most middle-class and lower-income Americans. Truly comprehensive health care reform was a cornerstone of his campaign pledge to reclaim "the American promise." Setting aside doubts, Obama would champion comprehensive health reforms, rather than nibbling at the edges of a broken health care system. Obama's decision to proceed after his election was made out of public view and, yet, it was a momentous decision; without it, comprehensive health reform would never have been pursued.

Full Speed Ahead

Once Obama decided that comprehensive health reform would be a top priority in year one, his White House team clicked into gear. When the President's first annual budget was issued on February 26, 2009, the document was boldly entitled "A New Era of Responsibility: Renewing America's Promise;" it laid out a blueprint for major reforms in health care, education, and energy, along with ongoing efforts to regulate and stimulate the economy. For health reform in particular, progressives and other Democrats anxious to hear that the President would move forward with comprehensive health reform in 2009 were delighted to learn that more than $630 billion was set aside as a "down payment." This was a serious "marker" in Washington parlance, indicating the President was putting money on the board to cover much (though not all) of what it would cost both to expand access and improve cost-effectiveness. In his speech introducing his budget blueprint, Obama claimed, "We are making a historic commitment to comprehensive health care reform. It's a step that will not only make families healthier and companies more competitive, but over the long term it will also help us bring down our deficit."[56]

By the time President Obama convened his first White House summit on health care reform on March 5, less than two months into his fledgling term, he had unambiguously signaled full speed ahead on his election promise to "make health care affordable for every single American." The decision made sense, as we have seen, but it was nevertheless high risk, because Obama was putting the prestige of his popular presidency on the line. Congressional deliberations would take an unforeseeable number of months, and the President would not be able to control the timing or outcomes. Knowing this, the President expressed no illusions that the coming legislative deliberations and maneuvers would be easy. Yet he seems still to have been hoping at that early juncture that he, as President, could help orchestrate a relatively broad consensus on strong but moderate legislation to achieve the twinned goals of access and affordability. That is why the White House summit assembled both Democratic and Republican leaders from Congress, and representatives from all kinds of major interest groups, not just unions and health care reformers aligned with Democrats, but also physicians groups, employers traditionally tepid or opposed to legislated health reforms, and insurers—all longtime ferocious foes of comprehensive change. The idea was to hear from everyone and look for solutions that would get as many on board as possible, and garner Republican as well as Democratic votes in Congress.

An open, bipartisan process was classic Obama—and of course central to the image of "rising above partisan rancor" that he had offered to American voters in the election. Obama had promised bold reforms—"change you can believe in"— along with bipartisanship. The signs so far in DC had not been promising about the prospect for combining these two, but Obama wanted to keep trying in health care.

At the March summit, the President and others were delighted when long-time crusader Senator Teddy Kennedy of Massachusetts, managed to come to the meeting and say a few inspiring words, at one of his last public appearances of any kind as he lost his battle with brain cancer. The mood at the White House summit was reported as unusually cooperative, and for a time afterward pundit opinion seemed to take it for granted that President Obama was right in projecting that some kind of comprehensive health reform, however difficult, would get "done this year"—2009.[57] Indeed, the Administration originally pushed for reform bills to get through both houses of Congress before the 2009 summer recess, with finally reconciled legislation ready for the President to sign well before Thanksgiving.[58]

A Mountain to Climb

The good feelings and high hopes that accompanied President Obama's wintertime affirmations that he would push ahead with comprehensive health reform would not last, and the hopeful timelines proved illusionary. In the end, the way reform would get done was anything but cooperative and bipartisan, and the process would drag on and on and on, trying everyone's patience, not least that of the watching American people. But before we tell the rest of the story, let us pause to note how high a mountain had to be climbed in 2009.

As we have learned, U.S. health care and approaches to paying for it for fortunate segments of the population were extremely complex on the eve of this latest attempt at bold reform. The reform challenge would be to squeeze enough savings out of an expensive system, and raise enough additional revenues through taxes and fees, to provide some sort of affordable health insurance to many millions of American citizens currently left without health insurance (undocumented immigrants and mere residents would still be left out). At the same time, reformers wanted to change the regulations for private health insurance and shift incentives and subsidies in the private and public health programs to protect the majority of Americans who were already insured as well as to encourage more efficient delivery of care. This was vital to reducing the rate of increase in costs, mitigating the burdens on families, businesses, and governments at all levels.

Yet, of course, "costs" in any system tend to be experienced by established interests as profits or entitlements to which they are accustomed. Thus, in U.S. health care as of 2008, the uninsured, or the inadequately insured, would appreciate major reforms such as expanded coverage or limits on insurance company abuses. But these potential beneficiaries and supporters tend to be young, lower-income, less educated, and not very political organized or powerful. On the other hand, many other interests or groups fearful of losses had a stake in the existing system, however broken. Would older Americans accept reductions in future spending on parts of Medicare, even if those cuts had little effect on their care, to help pay for expanded health insurance coverage? What would unionized workers or privileged executives and professionals think if someone wanted to tax, even slightly, their generous health benefits? Would all employers, not just those who already provide health benefits, be willing to pitch in? Would doctors and hospitals be willing to do more to care for patients without charging as much for treatments as in the past? And, of course, how would insurance companies and pharmaceutical giants react to new regulations that could reduce profits?

To ask all of these questions is virtually to answer them. Reform, no matter how carefully calibrated, would step on a lot of toes and arouse a lot of fears. As Obama and Democrats in Congress plunged ahead in 2009, opponents of health care reform—including Republicans who soon decided they did not want to let Obama win on this issue, either—could readily raise public worries and provoke costly lobbying and media efforts to push back against developing legislation. Comprehensive health reform in a mature, costly, patchwork system like the one in place in the early twenty-first-century United States is, indeed, a Sisyphean effort, where the boulder, if not pushed over the top, can fall back and crush many political lives.

2

THE YEAR OF PITCHED BATTLES: WHO FOUGHT FOR WHAT, WHY, AND HOW

Few Americans closely follow legislation as it inches through Congress. Life is too short and we have other important things to do. Headlines float by; talking heads yell at each other on TV; our Senator or Representative sends a newsletter explaining his or her position on a particularly touchy question. But mostly it is a blur, a hazy set of seemingly unrelated statements and votes that somehow, sometimes, culminate in a headline announcing a new law. If it is a big enough deal, a smiling president declares victory.

One of the oddities of the seemingly endless health reform battles that unfolded in and around Congress was the continuous media coverage. The usual blur became a bit more focused. Like the proverbial sausage factory that gets an intensive inspection, many Americans did not like what they heard and saw. As talk radio hosts and hard-edged television commentators decried the topsy-turvy journey of health reform through Congress, regular citizens reacted with anxiety—or anger—at unseemly deals, scary ads, and protracted maneuvering by ax-grinding groups and posturing legislators.

Most people tuned out at some point in the fall of 2009, concluding that nothing would come of all this—which might be just as well, because any actual results might not be good. Still, Congress sputtered along. On November 7, the House of Representative enacted a comprehensive health reform bill, the first time in history such a measure passed a chamber of Congress. This event only seemed to redouble the shouting and ominous ads on TV, and soon we were subjected to yet more protracted deal making in the Senate. With most Americans turning to holiday celebrations and speculation about which teams would make the NFL playoffs, the Senate went into endless sessions that Republicans denounced as a "power grab."

Appearing everywhere on television, Independent Connecticut Senator Joseph Lieberman executed his usual last-minute turns that make everyone angry, while Senate leaders scrambled to figure out something, anything, to attract his vote. Additional last-minute payoffs were negotiated among Democrats themselves, who hardly seemed to be on the same team. The "Louisiana purchase" had to be made to get Senator Mary Landrieu on board (with funds to offset the effects of Hurricane Katrina on health care funding). And the infamous "Cornhusker Kickback" was devised to send extra Medicaid subsidies to Nebraska in return for the vote of Senator Ben Nelson. In a midnight session on Christmas Eve, the Senate finally assembled just-enough votes to pass its own version of comprehensive health reform. But at what price? How worthwhile could the legislation be after all those special deals?

Washington, DC, insiders thought it was almost the end, that legislation finalized between the House and Senate would be on the President's desk before the end of the first month of the New Year. This was not to be, of course, and in chapter 3 we will see how reform almost died in January 2010, with the shocking victory of Republican Scott Brown in the Massachusetts special election to fill the Senate seat of Ted Kennedy, and required many weeks of emergency treatment to return to health. But in this chapter we probe the sausage-making factory that worked so hard, if undelectably, to produce the landmark House and Senate bills of late 2009. Who led the political maneuvers, and what deals were made to grease the path of reform? What was the impact of pressures from Tea Partiers on the right and progressive reform advocates on the left? What happened to hopes for bipartisanship? And what did everyone spend the year fighting about?

In spite of the fact that the process looked unseemly, it was not that different from what always happens when the U.S. government fashions major legislation, with drafting divided between the House and Senate, each chamber nudged by the White House and buffeted by interest groups and social movements. Despite the twists and turns of health reform's journey, it actually followed the paths and practices used for years by Republicans pressing for tax cuts, and by Democrats seeking to expand eligibility for government health care programs, such as Medicaid and the State Children's Health Insurance Program. Only the scope of the legislation was different this time, along with the 24/7 press coverage.

WHO LED THE CHARGE, AND WHAT TOOLS DID THEY HAVE?

A handful of critical players said the most colorful lines as the health reform drama staggered through its 2009 acts. The President and leaders in Congress were the colorful lead players, while others labored quietly but crucially behind the scenes.

Obama's Powers—and Their Limits

The newly elected, change-minded President Barack Obama naturally assumed center stage in lawmaking for health reform, though he was the lead in only a few scenes during 2009. He set the drama in motion, as we saw in chapter 1 by overruling some of his top advisors and proceeding with an attempt to orchestrate big, comprehensive health reforms amid the Great Recession. President Obama used his February 24, 2009, speech to Congress and the March 5 White House forum on health reform to outline the broad requisites of expanded access and cost controls that he wanted to see, while encouraging interest groups to come to the table with specific ideas, compromises, and contributions to paying the costs. Thereafter, the President set advisors to work on behind-the-scenes planning and bargaining, while urging committees in Congress to assemble the legislative specifics and the votes to pass bills. With Congress engaged in legislative sausage making, Obama spent much of 2009 as Cheerleader-in-Chief touring the country holding "town halls," featuring citizens or small business owners who needed help with affordable health care.

Obama had to take a more high-profile role when it looked as if forward momentum might stall. The congressional summer recess in August brought explosive antireform demonstrations by Tea Party activists, who mobbed public meetings that House and Senate members held with constituents back in their districts. Antireform demonstrations were, at times, marked by startling rhetoric—accusing Obama of being a Nazi or a Communist and claiming that health reform would set up "death panels" to decide on life or death for elderly Americans on Medicare. Vociferous protests coincided with ads attacking health reform from the Chamber of Commerce and other business interests. Opinion polls started to register growing worries in the general public about what reforms might mean for them personally. This always happens to public opinion when comprehensive legislation touching everyone's lives is debated in an angry way in DC and beyond; people start to think about what they might lose, rather than imagining gains for their families or the nation. Yet Democrats from Congress were surprised by the raucous town halls, and they were often bumbling in response. Would they begin to back off from reform when they returned from summer recess?

In addition, Obama was hearing again from doubters in his own White House. Just as at the critical juncture following the Inauguration when the President discussed whether to go forward with comprehensive health reform, advisors were getting cold feet—above all Obama's Chief of Staff

Rahm Emanuel.[1] He worried that, if Congress got spooked by public reactions, Obama (like Emanuel's former boss President Clinton, fifteen years before) could end up looking like a failed president if he pushed futilely for comprehensive reform. Why not back off into smaller gestures, like expanded health coverage for children and a few new rules about the private-health-insurance industry? As is his wont, Obama took valuable time to think this through—and some observers believe he missed chances for rapid and tough responses to gathering opposition from the Tea Partiers and business interests.[2]

But soon enough the President emerged from the valley of doubters to recharge the reform effort. He reportedly told Emanuel that he "had not been elected to do school uni-forms," a sharp riposte mocking the retreat into small efforts that Emanuel had helped Clinton make after his health reform plan fizzled in 1994.[3] With his White House team in order, Obama made a high-profile televised speech to a joint session of Congress on September 9, 2009, declaring "I am not the first president to take up this cause, but I am determined to be the last."[4] Obama's address reframed the debate as a clear-cut choice between doing something versus accepting a despised and unworkable status quo. Invoking the words of the recently deceased champion of health care reform, Ted Kennedy of Massachusetts, Obama elevated reform to a moral cause and conveyed a new sense of urgency to help people as well as the national economy. "Our collective failure to meet this challenge...has led to a breaking point....The time for bickering is over....Now is the time to deliver on health care."[5]

In this speech, as in earlier and later big addresses on health care, Obama did what an eloquent president can do best: focus public attention on a priority, corral wandering and wavering DC politicians, and signal gritty determination to vulture-like lobbyists circling Washington. The September speech slightly improved the standing of reform in national opinion polls, and nudged Congressional committees back to work. Specifically, Obama successfully prodded Congress toward, in due course, jumping three critical hurdles: first, getting a bill out of the one remaining Congressional committee that had not acted, the Senate Finance Committee, which would finally act on October 14, 2009; second, getting a majority for the House bill passed on November 7, 2009; and third, assembling a "super-majority" of 60 Senators to enact comprehensive reform in the Senate on Christmas Eve.

But if Obama's well-timed use of the "bully pulpit" was effective, let's not overestimate what a President can do, either with grand speeches or by issuing ultimatums. Throughout the health reform effort, pundits and commentators repeatedly criticized Obama for not doing more to force issues and push bold reform.[6] He was castigated for compromising away major features like the "public option," and for acquiescing in legislative deals like the "Cornhusker Compromise." As often happens when presidential behavior is assessed, Obama's supposed leadership failings were attributed to personal traits or flaws, such as his supposed worries about being seen as an angry black man or (as seasoned political reporter Elizabeth Drew put it) his "weakness" as exemplified in his "preference for consensus, his inclination to listen to all sides…, his occasional disinclination to take firm positions, his innate cautiousness…and his desire to please."[7]

In addition to calling for him to pound the table, critics wanted Obama to get specific much earlier on policy matters. They kept demanding that Obama "draw a line in the sand," that is, prod Congress and contending groups by saying what he would and would not accept in the final legislation that might reach his desk. When the two authors of this book did confidential interviews in Washington, DC, we found that key players *on all sides of contentious issues* were disappointed that the President had not jumped in to take public stands. Naturally, each actor wanted Obama to take his or her side and put those with whom each was arguing in their places.

Despite his proven oratorical abilities, the fact is that Barack Obama deliberately did *not* do at any point during 2009 what Bill Clinton did back at the very start of his own comprehensive health reform push in the fall of 1993: lay all his cards on the table. Back in 1993, President Clinton attempted to lead on health reform by devoting most of his first year in office to assembling a task force of over 500 experts to design a detailed plan to submit to Congress.[8] The effort provided a road map, but also ate up nine months, the early period of the president's popularity, and provided a big bulls-eye for opponents while irritating and sidelining Congressional committee chairs. As popular support for his health reform initiative waned a year into his presidency, President Clinton was begging committees in Congress to get moving—which they never did to any good effect. No legislation emerged from Congress before the Clinton plan fizzled.

This remembered history of "the last war" explains much of the reason why Obama and his advisors were determined to lead in a very different way, by having the President set broad guidelines with Congress charged to flesh out the details. Obama's decision to hand off the detailed work to Congress may have displeased pundits, but it freed him to concentrate on other huge emergencies—the economic crisis and the war in Afghanistan. And it allowed Congress to weave its ungainly way toward *actual legislation* by building the necessary coalitions to enact it through five committees and the entire House and Senate in less than a year. That amounts to lightening speed in DC time for big legislation.

There were prices to be paid by the President. Obama tried to keep Congress on a schedule, for example, by using a time-worn presidential technique, setting a deadline of July 2009, before the recess of Congress, for bills to pass the House and Senate. But the end of the session came and went, and the deadline was not met, not even close. Although four of the five committees had approved legislation, no action had been taken by the key Senate Finance Committee or either full chamber before that fateful recess with its Tea Party eruptions. The missed deadline intensified criticism of Obama's overly laid-back style. Another drawback of the President's above-the-fray, you-first-Congress approach was its discouraging impact on reform proponents, including the Organizing for America groups that continued from Obama's presidential campaign.[9] This activist network and others on the left of the Democratic Party wanted to push Congress on key measures. Obama's decision to remain at the level of broad principles stranded allies including liberal grass-roots forces for months at a time, leaving them to speculate about his detachment and reluctance to embrace fully a specific reform package. On balance, though, it is hard to fault the White House decision. There were bound to be trade-offs, yet Obama avoided the fate of Clinton and got legislation out of Congress.

During the months of legislative maneuvering on reform bills, moreover, a veritable army of Obama's aides were involved in quiet ways, as they tracked deliberations and provided technical assistance in testing and designing specific policies. We often equate the president with postcard photos of a small quaint building that we call the "White House." In truth, the staff of the executive office of the president has expanded over the past half century into hundreds of experts and aides housed in large office buildings around Washington. On health reform, Obama's Chief of Staff directed teams that worked with Congress in designing policy and keeping track of how organized groups and legislators were responding to different proposals as they were floated and discussed. With Senate leaders needing all sixty Democrats and Independents, Independent Senator Lieberman's warning of backpedaling on reform provisions on December 13, 2009, on a Sunday talk show produced a quickly scheduled meeting with a senior White House official. Similarly, concerns by Senator Dianne Feinstein about whether the expansion of insurance coverage would further strain California's already depleted budget produced a visit to her house (literally a "house call") by a top

White House official who camped out in the Senator's den for three hours to reassure her.[10] White House staff hovered on the edges of committee hearings and private sessions among legislators to convey the President's reactions and to collect intelligence on congressional discussions. Put simply, the President was a general of sorts, who brought many divisions to the battles over health reform.

Still, this overall look at President Obama's leadership tools and choices should remind us that no American president can dictate a legislative outcome, no matter how much swagger he brings to the challenge. A U.S. president is not like a British prime minister who (until the moment he or she loses a vote of confidence) commands a disciplined majority party in Parliament. The U.S. President as Commander in Chief can give orders that are routinely followed in foreign and national security policy, but in domestic affairs, the President can, at best, deploy aides and urge Congress to act. The constitutional system of checks and balances has long stymied presidents in domestic affairs.

There are considerations in the minds of Congress people more pressing than doing what the president asks. Each member of Congress wins "first past the post" majority elections, and responds to a distinct electorate in a particular district or state. In an area like health care, legislators routinely interact with businesses that do or do not offer insurance to employees; with hospitals and health providers worried about prices and regulations; with religious groups or unions determined to further their members' concerns; with constituents who vary by age, race, and insurance status. Legislators worry about where their campaign contributions and votes will come from, and they assess the impact of any legislation on the stakeholders and people who will provide these vital inputs to their political survival. Presidential prodding can go only so far in the face of local and regional specifics. Research shows the importance of constituent preferences—including the popularity of the president with constituents—as well as the party and ideological loyalties of legislators. Regional differences in economic and industrial economies also matter a lot and shape how representatives in Congress think about employment issues, social benefits including health insurance, and prices and profits and costs in the market arena.

Congressional Leaders and the Challenges They Faced

Indeed, if Congress is to do big things asked of it by a change-minded President like Obama, House and Senate leaders are vital in orchestrating voting coalitions. In this drama, leaders of Congress strutted the stage as much as the President and his aides, because they alone could shape the alliances and rally the majorities to get the bills passed.

The leader of the House of Representatives during 2009, the first woman to hold the position, was Nancy Pelosi, a liberal Democrat from San Francisco whose post as Speaker put her second in the line of presidential succession (after the Vice President). The highest-ranking female in U.S. political history, Pelosi has long been immersed in politics and is a masterful leader. Her father was a political powerhouse in Maryland as Baltimore's Mayor and Congressman, and she has developed, during her nearly quarter century in Congress, a steely resolve and pragmatic acceptance of the need to compromise to build majorities. By the time health reform arrived in the House, Pelosi enjoyed the respect of the 255 Democrats in her caucus—liberals, moderates, and conservatives alike. Renowned for hard work and attention to the tiniest details, she was in constant contact with her members and understood their individual concerns. Pelosi had a proven ability to shape and time legislation to "come to the floor" for a vote only when she was confident of a majority. She did not back off, and she did not lose when it came down to it.

Of course, as Speaker of the House, Pelosi enjoyed certain advantages according to established rules. The House proceeds by majority vote, and the minority party cannot delay bills for long. On the other hand, the entire 435-person membership of the House comes up for re-election every two years. Members are hypersensitive to the needs and moods of their constituents back home, and this means that a Speaker trying to rally majorities for controversial legislation must work very hard to find the "ideal point" that will garner more than 50% of the entire House without unduly hurting the reelection prospects of too many members of her party. Even with an unusually large Democratic majority in the 2009 House (which had 75 more Democrats than Republicans), Speaker Pelosi faced a huge challenge.

Pelosi's counterpart in the Senate was Majority Leader Harry Reid, a blunt-speaking Mormon from Nevada, whose job was considerably more difficult. A simple majority rules in the House, but Reid had to win 60 votes from 100 Senators of both parties to overcome what is known as the filibuster. This is a procedural maneuver that used to be only occasionally invoked, but now happens almost constantly; it allows opponents to delay or block action on legislation or on nominations of federal officeholders or judges. Individual Senators can slow things and trigger a potential filibuster by placing "holds"; any group of forty-one Senators can stop the progress of a bill altogether by refusing to vote to "cut off debate"—not that Senators actually have to talk all the time, or through the night. Years ago, the Senate devised insider-club practices to let everyone go home on time. Usually, those wanting to filibuster simply make the threat, and by current rule and custom, all progress on the legislation in question screeches to a halt without any further personal effort or any requirement that all forty-one filibuster supporters stand together in public.

During the first half of 2009, before the contested 2008 Senate election in Minnesota was resolved in the courts and Democrat Al Franken was seated in the summer, Senate Majority Leader Reid had fifty-seven Democratic Senators and two Independents who caucused with Democrats (the self-described socialist Bernie Sanders of Vermont, and the unpredictable Lieberman of Connecticut), and thus had to win over at least one Republican to break a potential filibuster. After Franken arrived, Reid could potentially move forward if he could unite all fifty-eight of the Democrats plus the two Independents—a situation that the press kept calling a "filibuster proof majority," but which, in fact, was a "super-majority" hurdle still very difficult to clear. After all, once the Democrats plus Independents apparently had sixty votes, Republicans were freed to engage only in nay-saying. The situation required Harry Reid to cater to the policy notions and personal whims of every single caucus member every day and every week and every month. (Pelosi, by contrast, enjoyed a seventy-five-seat majority and could pass bills by simple majority while still losing quite a few of her Democrats.)

As if things were not difficult enough, in addition to having to assemble supermajorities, the Senate Majority Leader is, by rule, less able than the Speaker of the House to control debate on the floor. A majority in the House dictates what bills are introduced on the floor, whether amendments can be offered, and how long they can be debated (if at all). By contrast, Senate rules empower each individual with substantial discretion to offer amendments. An open-ended amendment process, along with the filibuster, produces a potent weapon for the minority to slow or block majority efforts.

Harry Reid's ceaseless efforts to vault this daunting set of institutional hurdles proceeded as he personally faced a dire re-election challenge in 2010, with a steady stream of polls showing him trailing potential Republican opponents, some-times by double digits. Leading the charge for health reform in the Senate served the interests of the Democratic Party and sat-isfied Reid's personal desire to further important new policy for the nation. But the process was steadily and visibly alien-ating Nevada voters, already being hammered hard by the Great Recession. Reid persisted despite knowing that this might be his last hurrah in Congress.

Other Democratic leaders in Congress were vital throughout, including vote-counting deputies like the House Whip, Representative James E. Clyburn of South Carolina, and Deputy Senate Leader and Whip Dick Durbin of Illinois. We do not have space to go through all contributing players, but one additional Senator deserves specific discussion: the head of the Senate Finance Committee, Max Baucus of Montana. Baucus was pivotal to any prospect for health reform, in part because his committee controls taxes and spending, the life-blood of any major health reform. Even more important, Baucus had long-standing skill at cutting deals with business interests and articulating and accommodating moderate Senate Democrats, who not only weighed heavily in his own committee but were a powerful "swing" bloc in the Senate as a whole.

Of course, in a body with just 100 members, including a sixty-member Democratic/Independent caucus with no votes to spare, each centrist and left-leaning Democrat was also criti-cal (as liberals often reminded their colleagues). But in the hard-headed world of legislative bargaining, liberal Democrats ironically had *less* leverage when it came to brokering compro-mises, because they cared *more* about comprehensive health reform. Conservative and moderate Democrats cared, too, and most did not want to be the ones, as individuals, to defeat health reform and undermine Obama's presidency. But ideo-logical moderates and conservatives were more wary of expanding government powers in the health care economy. In a fix, they might walk away, or support only small changes, rather than accept liberal proposals they did not like or that offended their constituents or business interests to which they were oriented—proposals such as the public option in health insurance and generous subsidies for lower-income Americans (if those subsidies had to be paid for by taxes on employers or the rich). The most conservative Democrats could not only walk away from reform without angering most of their constit-uents; in some cases, such as Blanche Lincoln in Arkansas, they might actually do better in the next election by defying reform.

Liberals, on the other hand, wanted an expansion of governmental powers, and also had constituents, such as minorities, or the young, or liberal-minded professionals, who really wanted something big to pass. This created an imbalance in negotiations that disadvantaged the progressives and loaded the dice against liberal proposals. The bottom line was that liberal Democrats in Congress were willing to lose their battle for the public option in order to pass some version of comprehensive health reform. Everyone in the Senate Democratic caucus knew this—Max Baucus especially—so his Finance Committee was free to develop a bill that played down or omitted key liberal ideas.

As for Republicans in Congress, they were disadvantaged by having the smallest minority in decades. But their leaders could still use whatever rules were available to slow the legislative process, allowing interest groups opposed to reform to mount negative public campaigns. Republican leaders could also employ the bully pulpit to raise public concerns about Democratic plans for reform. These tactics were meant to rally Republican-base voters who were in opposition to legislation, and to complicate efforts by Pelosi and Reid to assemble majority or supermajority coalitions, especially when "Blue Dog" or conservative Democrats had to vote for reform despite fearful constituents back home. Following this oppositional game plan, Minority Leader John Boehner of Ohio—the GOP boss in the House—offered spirited public opposition, even though he lacked the power to obstruct Pelosi and the Democrats. Meanwhile, the rules of the game in the Senate allowed Republican leader Mitch McConnell of Kentucky to slow-walk health reform bills and amendments every step of the way, giving plenty of time over weeks and months for public reservations to percolate and trepidation to build in the Senate.

Most of all, McConnell and his Republican Senate colleagues compelled Reid and Democrats to walk a tightrope in assembling and holding the necessary sixty votes from the ranks of

Democrats and Independents alone. The result were pro-longed, publicly visible negotiating sessions that gave play to each preening Democratic Senator, with a back and forth, as concessions to one sent another into opposition. For example, concessions to Senators from regions with high medical costs might set off Senators from regions that delivered care effi-ciently and did not want to be punished for it in governmental reimbursement formulas. And concessions to liberals could prompt moderates to threaten to withraw from Reid's voting coalitions. Republicans cried "wolf" at each step, making normal legislative deal making visible to an increasingly anx-ious and bewildered public. This Republican tactic was espe-cially effective when individual Senators bargained for specific concessions for their state's businesses or citizens, or when Ben Nelson sought relief of Medicaid payments for his state's government. This sort of thing is fairly typical in Congress— and all the more so when a leader has no room for losing votes—because every single Senator can, in effect, hold up the entire body. But the deal making did not look good on national television.

As 2009 drew to a close and the Senate got ready to vote just before Christmas, many Americans had no idea that superma-jority votes are required to do anything at all in the Senate. (What private-sector business in America could work that way?) All most Americans understood or thought they saw was a bunch of Democrats making shady deals and failing to handle the nation's work very efficiently. Of course, that is exactly what Republican leaders wanted Americans to think; their unanimous opposition forced every Democrat to count and made health reform's legislative travails highly visible.

The Clout of the Bean Counters

Finally, we need to take note of some vital behind-the-scenes players, above all the interacting networks of experts and bean counters employed in the White House Office of Management and the Budget (OMB) and the Congressional Budget Office (CBO). The OMB houses the financial experts working for the President who help to shape his agenda, develop the budgets the President presents yearly to Congress, and figure out what presidential proposals will cost and what impact they will have on the deficit over time. The CBO was created by Congress to be their own impartial scorekeeper, staffed by nonpartisan experts charged with tallying up costs, figuring out revenue sources, and projecting budget impacts for bills making their way through the House and Senate. For some years, the fate of legislation in Washington, DC, politics has been heavily influenced by CBO "scores"—as the agency's estimates of fiscal footprints of bills are called in Washington-speak—because many fiscally cautious Representatives and Senators, including so-called Blue-Dog Democrats, will not support a bill unless it "costs out" in a way that does not blow up the federal deficit over the next ten to twenty years.

In a shrewd decision made out of public sight, well before 2009, Democrats concluded from the defeat of Clinton's 1993 proposal that the CBO was unavoidably a key player and that passing reform in the future would require adding new staff and expertise to accurately calculate costs and the impact of possible cost-saving measures in health care. The key figure was Peter Orszag, appointed CBO director after the Democrats regained their majorities in 2006. A major Orszag priority was to prepare CBO's "intellectual groundwork" by hiring more staff and strengthening its capacity to cost out a stream of health proposals to keep pace with an ongoing legislative process.

Tellingly, once Obama was elected President, he moved immediately to appoint the same Peter Orszag as Director of the OMB in his White House.[11] This would enable Obama's team to work closely with legislators to develop technically sound proposals that stood a chance of scoring well at CBO. Without the CBO groundwork after 2006 and the transfer of Orszag's policy planning and accounting capacities to the

Obama White House in 2009, calculations about the budgetary specifics and future impact of health reform ideas might well have been more hit-and-miss, not to mention even more protracted than they always are, perhaps tripping up the drive to health reform.

Although the CBO had, in place, enhanced capacities, it was and is a nonpartisan agency fiercely determined to guard its independence and expert impartiality. The CBO shrouds its internal workings in secrecy, shares official results simultaneously with both political parties and the public, and keeps its own counsel on how measures are scored. Thus, when Democrats pressed for private preliminary scores to test different packages in 2009, the CBO refused to work in a partial way, and continued to update and follow the published rule book that catalogues its methods.[12] Moreover, the 2009 CBO did not always score some cost-saving measures as generously as the White House and Congressional Democrats expected, repeatedly leaving them to scramble to come up with additional ways to hold down long-term costs in health care. A striking indication of the independent clout of the CBO was the relief, elation, even pleasantly shocked surprise with which House and Senate leaders greeted favorable long-term budget projections for health reform bills issued in late 2009 and early 2010. Those conclusive CBO scores, which were key to holding majority voting coalitions, had been awaited with hope and dread. Famously, Senate Whip Dick Durbin quipped "That's what it's going to say on my tombstone: 'He was waiting for C.B.O.' "[13]

DEALS WITH THE DEVIL? INSIDER BARGAINS WITH HEALTH CARE STAKEHOLDERS

Legislating for health reform dragged out over many months because lawmakers could not just sit down with experts and write the finished product. Endless consultations had to take place and many bargains had to be worked out among interest groups and within each house of Congress. Such bargains and "deals" are, for many Americans, an unsavory part of politics. Why don't the politicians just do right by the people? But in the world as it is, those devising major new legislation have to get down in the weeds. There was no way to reform one-sixth of the U.S. economy without engaging the major economic stakeholders, especially health care providers, pharmaceutical companies, and private insurers.

Why Reformers Bargained

Health reform as devised by liberals and moderates in the present day United States is filled with paradoxes. Critics may loudly denounce a "government takeover," but actually Democratic Presidents from Carter through Clinton to Obama have set aside, from the get-go, the notion of a single payer system like the one enjoyed since the 1970s by our neighbors to the North. Canadians personally choose doctors and hospitals just like U.S. people do, but one payer, the government in each province, negotiates and pays the bills, instead of having hundreds of different kinds of insurance forms to fill out, plus intertwined bureaucracies run by insurance companies and government to process the forms and collect the payments. Single-payer advocates in the United States believe it would save a lot of money and time to have this system here, too, and in recent years, many doctors, exasperated by filling out forms all day and by being second-guessed by insurance agents, have come around to this position. But for moderate U.S. health reformers, including elected Democratic officials, a single-payer system is not realistic. They feel that reforms have to start with what the United States already has in place and nudge things forward from there.

Mainstream reformers have been determined to work with the mixed public-private system, protecting and regulating private insurance while using existing government programs and modest subsidies to help Americans of modest means gain coverage. Perhaps not surprisingly, stakeholders in the market economy applaud this basic approach, particularly provisions that might lower costs for employers or generate more paying customers for private insurers, pharmaceutical companies, and for-profit providers. In other words, the so-called government takeover is no such thing; it is a set of changes in taxes, subsidies, and regulations cheered on by significant elements of the private sector.

Equally paradoxical is the double game that mainstream Democrats play. They publicly campaign against the so-called selfishness and abuses of private-health-economy stake-holders, but at the same time include them in policy discussions and seek to forge bargains behind the scenes. In 2009, pivotal bargains were struck behind closed doors in which reformers gave concessions worth billions of dollars and, in return, many (but not all) of the market stakeholders agreed to support reform or withhold vocal opposition. To be sure, there were important business groups that vociferously countered Obama and the Congressional Democrats—most importantly, the Chamber of Commerce that devoted millions to running negative ads, and the National Federation of Independent Businesses that claims to speak for small businesses and is especially attuned to employers who do not offer insurance to employees. However, many other business associations and major corporations were willing to play ball to varying degrees.

Without fully judging backroom deals, we should try to comprehend why and how they happened. Some liberal advocates outside government were infuriated and baffled by the insider deals, and equally exasperated with the failure of Democrats to go all out in using government powers to expand public insurance and regulate drug prices. For example, Jane Hamsher, founder of the liberal Web site Firedoglake, decried the sweetheart deals and, especially, the pact with drug makers as a betrayal of "what Obama ran on" and as "sacrificing...something really good."[14] This sort of backlash was anticipated by Obama and senior Democratic leaders of

Congress, but they nevertheless held to a simple hard-headed conclusion about their relationship with the economically hefty stakeholders: no (uneasy) peace, no reform.

Having witnessed the demise of Clinton's reform effort, Obama's team accepted that major economic-interest groups with profits at stake would be much more vigilant, motivated, and organized than the diffuse public that would benefit from reforms. Patients abused by insurers, low-income working people who are uninsured, and middle-class Americans facing rising costs and receding coverage—all of them would lack the clout and resources to loudly and effectively promote beneficial changes. Cutting deals with potential knock-out opponents was seen by Democrats in office as a necessary strategy for dampening and dividing opposition while a new framework for health insurance was put in place. Public leverage could then be further strengthened in future years. This was their game plan and they stuck to it.

White House Chief of Staff Rahm Emanuel and Senate Finance Committee Chair Max Baucus took the lead in developing and following a coordinated game plan to (as the *New York Times* put it) "keep powerful groups at the table [and]...prevent them from allying against [Obama] as they did against Clinton." Along with other administration officials, the White House's political guru, David Axelrod, made it clear that accommodations to stakeholders were the price of "get[ting] things done within the system as it is."[15] There was "no chance at winning the necessary 60 votes in the Senate if interest groups were against you," explained a White House aide.[16] An aide to a senior Senate Democrat closely involved in the outreach elaborated that negotiations were used to induce "every stakeholder in discussion to keep talking" and to prevent or even delay them from attacking the bill.[17] Inside players discounted liberal criticism as "underestimat[ing] the strategic value of...alliances in...being able to keep [the reform] thing going."[18] Indeed, the staff of liberal icon Ted Kennedy also participated in the outreach to the stakeholders to forestall an early and sustained "massed attack" and to "keep them at the table" in order to "road test ideas," detect fault lines, and convey the "sense of being listened to," as possible compromises were devised. Looking back at the deal making and its impact in passing legislation in the Senate, a senior Kennedy aide bluntly concluded that "without a shadow of doubt the accommodations were necessary...."[19]

How Were Deals Struck?

In committee hearings and dozens of private sessions, senior government officials explored with insurers, medical providers, drug manufacturers, employers, unions, and others the effects of different reform packages. Many changes were made in legislation in response to the feedback. Nothing really surprising happened; this is how government typically conducts its consultations in Democratic and Republican eras alike.

Deal making also entailed bartering with interests who make a living in the health industry and whose bottom lines are impacted. The White House and senior Democrats from Congress had candid, bottom-line conversations laying out "how much the stakeholders stood to gain" in exchange for their willingness to "mute their opposition and outcry"—as an influential congressional staffer explained.[20] Although each major type of stakeholder got a specially tailored deal, the Democrats' main approach was to stress the bottom-line benefits of 32 million new paying customers.

Health care providers were told that reform would pay big—$171 billion for hospitals and $228 billion for doctors—and in turn the American Hospital Association agreed to accept $155 million less in Medicare payments over ten years, while the American Medical Association (AMA) consented to future payment reductions that amounted to $80 billion.[21] The AMA's buy-in was particularly striking because it had been the implacable foe of national health insurance reform for nearly a century, including its opposition to the enactment of Medicare back in 1965 when it threatened to go on strike and refuse to treat ill patients. Although it dropped its historic opposition and supported even the November 2009 House legislation, the most liberal bill to pass Congress, the AMA did not get all it wanted in the end. Legislators refused to permanently eliminate scheduled cuts in Medicare's payment formula for doctors, and the Senate adopted an independent commission on Medicare payments, which the AMA fears may be less responsive than Congress to AMA pressure in the future.

The *big drug companies* are taken care of by a powerful lobbying group known as PhRMA (Pharmaceutical Research and Manufacturers of America, pronounced "Farma") led during this episode by the flamboyant, back-patting former congressman Billy Tauzin. A man who relishes deal making, Tauzin struck a bargain to charge lower drug prices and pay fees that amounted to $85 billion over ten years, in exchange for a true windfall for his industry—tens of billions of dollars in new customer prescriptions from the newly insured and from "filling in the doughnut hole" to improve Medicare's prescription drug subsidies.[22] Big PhRMA also got rules protecting them against new competition from makers of cheaper generic drugs (specifically biologic medications), as well as a commitment that Obama would not support importation of cheaper medications from other countries, even though he had made such a promise to voters during the 2008 campaign.[23] The deal between Tauzin and the White House and key Democrats made people on all sides angry. Many rank-and-file Democrats in Congress condemned what they considered unjustifiable giveaways and fought to change the deal in the public's favor. But the White House and Senate leaders blocked those efforts, while Tauzin pumped $100 million in advertising and other efforts to pass reform.[24] Some drug companies protested that Tauzin conceded too much and, according to speculation in Washington, forced him out in early 2010.

Private health insurance companies are the most intriguing and misunderstood negotiator with Democratic reformers. Rhetoric from Obama and leading Democrats flared up against abusive insurance companies from time to time, but these verbal attacks masked the extensive negotiations that the White House and senior figures in Congress had with insurers during 2009, with repeated efforts made toward reaching an agreement. Not long after Obama's inauguration, private negotiations began in earnest with insurers and its lobbyist arm, America's Health Insurance Plans (or "AHIP"), whose President and CEO, Karen Ignagni, participated in the President's health care summit in March 2009 and declared "our commitment to play, to contribute, and to help pass health-care reform this year."[25] Ignagni also signed onto a letter to Obama offering to reduce insurance prices and costs voluntarily.[26] In the early fall of 2009, moreover, the Senate Finance Committee rejected what insurers most intensely opposed—the public option—and adopted forty-eight amendments that responded to insurance industry complaints, provoking Senator Rockefeller to quip that "the insurance industry is not running this markup but it is running certain people in this markup."[27] (A *markup* is what committee members do to finalize provisions and fine-tune language in a bill; lobbyists take a keen interest in such nitty-gritty, because it is where the rubber often meets the road in government regulation of the economy. As we show in the final chapter, these quiet concessions are now being exploited by insurers and other special interests, as the new health reform law is put into practice.) In addition to such concessions, insurers were closely calculating their return on potential future expansions of subsidized insurance coverage, and were encouraged by press reports in September 2009 that Democrats had "already agreed to grant one of the [insurance] industry's dearest wishes: a requirement that everyone have coverage."[28] This was the so-called individual mandate for every American to buy insurance, with government help to make it affordable—obviously a profit-generating dream for private insurers.

Deal making with insurers sharply deviates from the public image of Democrats attacking private insurers and insurers running ads that warned against "government takeovers."[29] In truth, Democrats accepted that private insurers would continue to dominate health care financing and strained to cut a deal with them; and for their part, the insurers welcomed certain types of significant government intervention. It is telling what ultimately prompted insurers to move into aggressive opposition to Obama and bills developing in Congress: the September decision of the Senate Finance Committee—under pressure from Republicans—to weaken the planned penalties for Americans who, after 2014, do not obtain insurance. This weakening of the individual mandate worried private insurers, because they feared that new reform regulations would force them to take all patients regardless of health conditions, whereas insignificant penalties for people choosing not to buy insurance would allow a lot of younger Americans to skip coverage. In that scenario, the companies' profit margins would decline. Note the irony: Despite its ads and public criticisms of too much government, insurers muffled its opposition when it looked as if draft legislation would impose an individual mandate with teeth, but then moved into public opposition to health care reform overall when they "worried that the penalties are too low or will not be enforced," possibly reducing their ultimate pool of paying customers to "only" 94% of Americans![30] Too little government was what moved insurers into open revolt. This is one of many instances in which rhetoric about big government should be taken with a grain of salt and deserves a closer look.

Insurers moved into vigorous open opposition in October 2009 by issuing a commissioned study from Price Waterhouse Cooper charging that health reform would produce massive increases in premiums for insured middle-class Americans.[31] The accounting firm acknowledged that it had been instructed

by AHIP to leave out the effect of subsidies that offset the premium hikes as well as some cost-reducing parts of reform bills.
In a loud warning shot back across the bow, reformers
responded immediately and with full force to demonstrate to
insurers (and other stakeholders) the cost of opposition, of
backing away from bargains and negotiations. The day after
the insurers' report was issued, the White House set up a "war
room" to "shred" it, to attack its credibility with the press and
public.[32] Independent analysts closely examined the study
from Price Waterhouse Cooper and, as the exaggerations by
insurers were exposed, Price Waterhouse Cooper distanced
itself from the claims of insurers. Not only did insurers become
a whipping post for reformers, regulations of insurance practices that had been in the works were tightened—for instance,
the practice of attracting the healthy and avoiding the ill or
charging them substantially more in premiums was ended.

As stakeholder deals were struck (or attempted), the broad
public, for the most part, lacked similarly organized and influential brokers. A partial exception was AARP, which has
grown from its founding in 1958 into a 40 million member
organization that lobbies for Americans of fifty years of age
and over. AARP stood to gain from the expansion of paying
customers who might choose to buy their lucrative supple-
mental insurance programs for older people; and the organization also strongly favored expansion of Medicare's
prescription drug benefit to cover the so-called doughnut
hole—the gap between $2,700 when coverage stopped (as of
2009) and $6,154 when it kicked in again. Millions of senior
citizens faced very high costs within that coverage gap. As
legislation took shape that improved various Medicare benefits, including subsides to close the gap in prescription coverage, AARP became a stalwart supporter of reform including
the House version enacted in November.[33]

All in all, the deals with stakeholders paid the anticipated
political dividends to the White House and Democrats
advancing bills in Congress. Not only did the descendants of

many of the most rabid stakeholder opponents of reform in 1993–1994 reverse or muffle their positions in 2009; some of them actually contributed to ad campaigns promoting reform. Aides to Obama and Baucus convened meetings in Democratic Party offices to launch a new consortium of interest groups—Americans for Stable Quality Care—that financed millions of dollars of advertisements to promote reform.[34] In the first six months after Obama's Inauguration, the groups favoring and opposing reform spent $57 million on television ads, with the advocates outspending the critics.[35] Opposition ads grew stronger later in the year of legislative debates, but Obama and the Democrats never did have to suffer the full force of all-out, unified business opposition.

OUTSIDE PRESSURES FROM RIGHT AND LEFT

As inside bargains were struck, outside public pressures were also brought to bear on Congress and the White House. Pressures came from longstanding interest groups, to be sure; and from media commentators trying to fill a 24/7 news cycle. Yet, as often happens when something really big is at stake in Congress, widespread and loosely interconnected grass-roots movements raised their voices and made a difference. Tea Partiers and other populists were active on the right, demanding the outright defeat of reform, while progressives worked through labor unions and alliances of reform advocates to bring pressure from the left on behalf of favored provisions they wanted in final legislation—above all a "public option" to let working-age Americans choose government-funded health insurance like Medicare. Popular pressures on Congress thus came from both directions and met at the ideologically charged flash point of the federal government's direct role in health insurance.

Millions of Americans were put on edge at the end of 2008 and in early 2009 by the financial rescues of Wall Street and big auto companies pushed through by outgoing President George

W. Bush, followed by the federal "stimulus" bill, the American Recovery and Reinvestment Act, ushered into law by newly inaugurated President Obama. Among populists on the right, Washington's "big spending" (conflating the stimulus and earlier bailouts as one and the same) fueled a ferocious backlash against the federal government, denounced as threatening to raise taxes and intrude on local and personal freedoms. Meanwhile, self-styled progressives, on the left of the Democratic Party, wanted more federal government activism to rein in corporate abuses. The Wall Street financial meltdown and ensuing Great Recession confirmed progressives' longstanding belief that big corporations, including health care stakeholders, are out to squeeze ordinary Americans. In short, putting comprehensive health reform forward during 2009 was like waving a red flag in front of angry groups on the right and left.

"Just Say No" Outcries from the Right

For grassroots conservatives, health reform was the latest and perhaps greatest threat of government expansion. The conservative backlash against health reform was stirred up by cable television and Fox talk show host Sean Hannity. Further egged on by Rush Limbaugh's withering attacks, conservative anger gained expression via a wide-ranging set of organizations— from local Republican Party chapters and conservative advocacy groups like Freedom Works to the loosely organized clusters of Tea Party protesters who listened to Fox News and often used Internet devices such as MeetUp to get together locally and act on their grievances. A *New York Times* survey, taken not long after health reform passed in 2010, revealed that 90% of Tea Party supporters disapproved of Obama's handling of the issue, believing that the President had expanded government too much and was moving the country toward socialism.[36] (These reactions were far more oppositional than the country overall—the same poll found, for instance, that

Obama's handling of health reform was criticized by 51% of the general public.) This survey also found that Tea Party participants and sympathizers, around 25% of the overall population, are older, richer, and whiter than Americans in general, and have voted overwhelmingly for Republicans in the past. Tea Partiers are, in essence, the most conservative and angriest members of the long-term Republican base. They also hold views on race and immigration considerably more negative toward nonwhites than the views other citizens, including other Republicans.

Tea Party supporters and backers of Congressman and 2008 GOP presidential candidate Ron Paul—a libertarian who favored substantially reducing government—became shock troops in opposing health reform. During the August 2009 congressional break, Sean Hannity's Web site exhorted visitors to "Become Party of the mob!" by attending town hall meetings held by their member of Congress. The Web site of Tea Party Patriots advised visitors to "pack the hall" and "Yell out and challenge the Representative's statements early" to "get him off this prepared script." This fiery opposition burst onto the national scene when Republican congressman Joe Wilson startled even Republican leaders by his breach of protocol when he shouted, "You lie!" to President Obama during his September speech; Wilson was seeking to register his disagreement with the President's claim that pending health reform bills would not allow coverage to illegal immigrants.

Ironically, a lot of Tea Partiers and other conservatives are older men and women on Medicare, which is of course a health insurance program that is fully funded and run by the government. But they see Medicare as a benefit they have earned in lifetimes of hard work, so their participation in this socialized program does not, in their thinking, contradict strong opposition to *other* government social programs, such as expanded Medicaid or the public option. Conservatives railed against parts of health reform intended to cover younger and less affluent Americans, denouncing these not just as "government takeovers" but also as "handouts" to people who have not earned the benefits.

Progressives Draw Lines in the Sand

On the left, no organizations matched the publicly visible and vivid efforts of aroused conservatives, in part because no television station played the exhorting role on the left that Fox did on the right, but also because progressives were already organized prior to 2009 in a series of labor unions and advocacy groups that were not "news" to the mainstream media.

Liberals who wanted comprehensive health care reform started forming alliances and planning to push the White House and Congress well before the 2008 election. Like everyone else in the broad Democratic Party orbit, grass-roots progressive organizations tried to learn from "what went wrong" back in 1993–1994. Key liberal advocacy groups and foundations and funders encouraged planning ahead this time, believing that progressives were not prepared back in 1993.[37] What is more, this time around in the long-running quest for universal health insurance in America, most liberal health care reformers decided in advance that they would not insist on the single-payer approach, but would, instead, champion a compromise idea called the "public option," a proposal to create a publicly run health insurance plan to compete side by side with private health insurance.[38] Having compromised this much, however, self-styled realist progressives did not want a Democratic President and Congress to compromise any more with private health insurance companies. True health reform must, they felt, include a public insurance plan as one choice—to "keep insurance companies honest" and provide nonelderly citizens with affordable care that did not include profits for private insurers and bonuses for insurance executives.

During 2009, as conservatives were trying to stop health reform altogether, most progressives exerted targeted pressure on committees of Congress and on the White House at critical junctures, when reform stood on the precipice of failure or there was a likelihood of substantial backtracking from progressive tenets. MoveOn.org and other liberal groups were active, but the chief orchestrator of pressure was Health Care for America Now (or HCAN).[39] HCAN brought together more than one thousand organizations (including prominent liberal and labor groups) to press for the public option to be included in House and Senate bills. HCAN and other progressive groups also pushed for better subsidies to help needy Americans buy insurance. And the unions within this overall alliance pressed hard against one alternative for helping to pay for health reform—the so-called Cadillac tax that imposed an excise tax on the most expensive employer-provided health plans. Most highly generous employer health plans cover executives and managers, but some had been earned by unionized workers in mines and other blue-collar jobs in exchange for salary increases over many years. Determined not to lose their hard-won gains, unions with the best insurance coverage were determined not to let either the White House or Democrats in Congress trim them back. The progressive alliance backed unions on this issue, miffed that DC Democrats would be going against the wishes of their most loyal organized supporters.

In their principal campaign for the public option, progressives had many Americans on their side in a general way. National opinion polls repeatedly showed sizeable majorities supporting a public option, ranging from over 60% at one point to somewhat smaller percentages, but still majorities, as public perceptions of the overall reforms at issue became more negative.[40] Precisely because public opinion seemed enabling, many public option champions on the left were enraged by the inability or unwillingness of the White House to join with progressives in Congress to deliver the public option—presumably on the theory that demands from Obama could have persuaded the likes of Senators Lieberman, Nelson, and Lincoln to go along. Adam Green, a founder of Progressive

Change, complained that Obama's Chief of Staff had a "loser mentality" that led him to be "afraid of a fight" and rely on a "very, very risk-averse" approach, urging "the President to cave instead of fighting for real change."[41] Liberal *New York Times* columnist Paul Krugman hammered Obama, not even six months in office, for "search[ing] for common ground where none exists" and negotiating "with himself" for "policies that are far too weak." Zeroing in on Obama's unwillingness to endorse a public option, Krugman derided him for delivering a "gratuitous giveawa[y] in an attempt to sound reasonable" and warned that "reform isn't worth having if you can only get it on terms so compromised that it's doomed to fail."[42] As conservatives ambushed town hall meetings, Krugman recoiled at Obama's "deer-in-the-headlights" reaction to "unreasoning, unappeasable opposition" and questioned whether he had the fortitude and leadership skill to "rise to the challenge."[43]

Despite pressure and anguish from the left, the dickering with moderate Democratic Representatives left only a watered down and weak public option in the November 2009 House legislation—the most liberal health reform to pass in Congress. What the House approved would never have been available to more than a tiny portion of Americans: the CBO estimated that the House version would have reached only 2% of the insured after reform is fully implemented, that is, 3 to 4 million people out of 200 million nonelderly expected to have insurance.[44] That was the high water mark for the public option; even weaker versions fell short of the sixty votes needed to overcome the filibuster in the Senate (exactly how far short is a matter of dispute, but we think a weak public option could have gained, at best, fifty-two votes from liberal and moderate Senators). In time, many progressive advocates had to face the precariousness of finding sufficient like-minded allies inside Washington's inhospitable institutions. As Democrats in Congress cobbled together majorities in nail-biting cliffhangers in the fall of 2009, many initial supporters of the public option grudgingly accepted that it would not be possible to pass a meaningful plan that included it, at least during this round of reform.

What Did Outside Pressures Accomplish?

Did the progressive focus on the public option hurt reform prospects? Certain DC Democrats and some reform promoters complained that public option advocates were risking the defeat of the entire reform package by keeping it "always in the room," when the focus should have been on enacting legislation before the end of 2009. President Obama chided "my progressive friends" in his September speech to a joint session of Congress for losing track of the goal—insurance reform and universal coverage—in favor of seeking the public option, which Obama called "only a means to that end."[45] Republican Senator Grassley, a member of the Senate Finance Committee, singled out the public option as a "major impediment to getting a bipartisan agreement."[46] And Democratic fashioners of bills in the Senate derided public option supporters for mistakenly assigning it "Ptolemaic value."[47] A lifelong advocate of national health insurance professed to being "mad at the left" for insisting on the public option in the Senate to the detriment of important and feasible enhancements that would improve the lives of millions of Americans—from strengthening the rules governing insurance exchanges to expanding subsidies for lower-middle-income people.[48]

Our assessment of the impact of progressive advocacy, particularly for the public option, is calmer in retrospect. That advocacy may always have been doomed to fall short, given the realities of interest-group bargains and coalition building in the Senate. Tenacity may have passed into self-defeating gestures at certain critical junctures late in the process when reform hung in the balance. Nonetheless, pressure from progressives kept the public option in play long after real-politic-minded Democrats, including the White House, would have brushed it aside. This, in turn, meant that, when the endgame eventually came in each chamber of Congress, the more liberal Democratic Senators could say that they needed *other* provisions supported by progressives in return for dropping the public option. This dynamic almost resulted in allowing an expanded buy-in to Medicare for Americans 55–64 years old, a very popular provision meant to substitute for the public option that Harry Reid dropped only when Senator Lieberman (who had previously claimed to support this compromise) refused at the eleventh hour to accept it. Even so, liberals won higher taxes on the rich and more generous subsidies for lower- and middle-income Americans than they might otherwise have done, especially in the House bill and to a degree in the final Senate bill. As Peter Dreier summed up the inside-and-outside dynamic on the center left, progressive "activism on the ground" created pressure for bolder reforms and gave "liberal elected officials more room to maneuver."[49]

Tea Partiers on the right also made a difference from the outside. Because they were mobilized and intensely focused potential voters for the GOP, Tea Partiers and other right-wing activists were a large part of the reason Republicans in Congress would not visibly engage or formally compromise as health reform bills progressed, driving the breakdown in visible bipartisanship we are about to discuss. Conservative populist mantras to "just say no" meant that any Republican Representative or Senator inclined to bargain with Democrats for specific health bill provisions that, from his or her perspective, could improve legislation and possibly justify voting for a reform bill, would likely face an angry base electorate in looming primaries. This could easily mean defeat for Republican incumbents at the hands of right-wing opponents in their own party, and they knew it.

WHAT HAPPENED TO BIPARTISANSHIP?

Media pundits with their eyes on DC talk incessantly about the value of "bipartisan compromise," defined as public support and official votes from members of both parties for major leg-islation. Partly, this is just an inside-the-Beltway obsession, but it also represents an aspiration shared by many voters—and espoused by Barack Obama himself during the 2008 election campaign, when he repeatedly promised to fix the broken system in Washington, DC, by promoting dialogue and drawing ideas to address national problems from Republicans and Democrats alike. During the health reform debates, the President gave every appearance of trying to carry through. He convened White House forums that included groups and politicians of all stripes, urged Republican leaders in Congress to offer proposals and amendments, and invited key Republican moderates like Senator Olympia Snowe of Maine for repeated tête-à-têtes in the Oval Office. Most telling, to the exasperation of many liberals in his party, the President spent crucial weeks and months in the middle of 2009 deferring to the efforts of Senate Finance Committee Chair Max Baucus to produce a bill supported by at least two or three Republicans. If this could be done, the President seemed to think, it would turn health care reform into a bipartisan endeavor, not just a Democratic Party project.

With White House encouragement, Baucus actually side-lined most of his twenty-three-member committee and con-vened a special caucus, called the "Gang of Six," to see if three hand-picked Democrats (himself along with New Mexico Senator Jeff Bingaman and North Dakota Senator Kent Conrad) could find common ground with three Republicans (Wyoming Senator Mike Enzi, Maine Senator Olympia Snowe, and Baucus's longtime personal friend, and the ranking Republican, Iowa Senator Chuck Grassley). If this Gang of Six had been able to write a bill that all were committed to vote for, that would probably have changed the entire dynamic. The Senate Finance Committee and then, perhaps, the Senate as a whole might have been prodded by Baucus and the President to go along with whatever emerged, setting up a tense endgame of negotiations to compromise a more liberal House bill written by Democrats with a Senate bill significantly tilted toward conservative and business preferences by Republicans.

More than half a year was devoted to substantive bipartisan discussions and negotiations by the Gang of Six, closeted from time to time with staff from the White House and the CBO. Only a few months after Obama's inauguration, Baucus and his staff were meeting with the lead Republican, Chuck Grassley, to present options and an outline of legislation.[50] And for his part, Grassley presented—over the trepidations of his staff and his own political instincts—several provisions the GOP would later attack, including the mandate requirement that every individual obtain insurance, reductions in future Medicare spending, and substantial spending on subsidies to allow the less affluent to purchase insurance. There were several dozen one-on-one in-depth sessions between Baucus and Grassley as well as thirty-one meetings of the Gang of Six. Senators and staff in these meetings confirm Grassley's later description of them on the Senate floor as driven by the shared conviction that "something has to be done...[and that] [w]e worked for a long period of time, thinking we could have something bipartisan."[51]

As it turned out, though, the Gang of Six process, after repeated delays—which, in retrospect, the White House would regret[52]—never reached fruition. Senator Grassley broke from his old friend Max Baucus and started denouncing "Democrat" health reform by late summer, going so far as to suggest that "death panels" might be in the emerging bills, a ridiculous lie popular with angry right-wing activists even though the supposedly offending provision for voluntary end-of-life consultations was proposed by a conservative Republican Senator.[53] Only one Republican Senator, Olympia Snowe, voted for the Senate Finance bill reported out in October—and she soon backed out of further Senate deal making and joined all other Republicans in supporting a filibuster to prevent final Senate actions and opposing the Christmas Eve Senate enactment of comprehensive reform.

This was the publicly visible, official dynamic: dying possibilities for any cross-party cooperation on health reform. Yet in the details of reform provisions hashed out in the Gang of Six as well as in other committees and staff deliberations, the story was more complicated. Hundreds of amendments proposed by House or Senate Republicans received enough bipartisan support to make it into advancing legislation, and (as we will see further in the final section of this chapter) many concrete ideas about how to expand access or control costs came from Republican sources.[54] Significant elements of the final legislation that the President ended up signing in 2010 were shaped by these negotiations. Officially, though, Republicans would not take public credit for health reform bills or vote for them.[55] This lack of formal support from Republicans is without historic parallel in major U.S. social policy making since the New Deal, and raises the question of what was going on.

A large part of the answer lies at the level of simple electoral calculation. Republican leaders were, just like their Democratic counterparts, thinking back to the 1993–1994 episode of failed comprehensive health reform. Where Democrats sought to correct for the mistakes they thought were made back then (by devising better presidential, legislative, and advocacy tactics to turn failure into success this time around), Republicans hoped to repeat the political and electoral triumphs their party had enjoyed in 1994 by, yet again, defeating a major Democratic push for comprehensive health reform. Firebrand South Carolina Republican Senator Jim DeMint proclaimed in July 2009 that if "we" Republicans "are able to stop Obama on [health reform], it will be his Waterloo. It will break him." Using less inflammatory language, GOP Senate leader McConnell openly discussed his plan to "uni[fy his partisans] behind [the calculation]…that they stand to gain politically in next year's elections if Democrats do nothing."[56] "It was absolutely critical," McConnell openly counseled Senate Republicans, "that everybody be together [to prevent Democrats from being]…able to say it was bipartisan" and thus "convey to the public that this [is] O.K."[57] Using polls, McConnell offered loaded words and catchphrases to attack Democrats and attract Republican and Independent voters by invoking the threats of rising "government spending," "debt," and "bailouts."[58] "[T]he reward for playing team ball," he confidently explained, was "the reversal of the political environment and the possibility that we will have a bigger team next year."[59]

Individual Republicans who cared about policy substance and showed some willingness to negotiate with Democrats in the Gang of Six or other venues were confronted and pressured by party leaders McConnell and Boehner, leaders who were—as Senator Grassley put it—"very concerned about…the directions the policy discussions were taking."[60] In short, any compromises would undermine the Republican Party's effort to make big gains in 2010 and 2012.

Another problem, of course, was that would-be bipartisan negotiators like Chuck Grassley in the Finance Committee were more willing to intellectually entertain possible compromises than they were able or willing to deliver actual votes. Republican Grassley and Democrat Baucus were long-time personal friends and—with perhaps a touch of romantic rosy retrospect—both leaders and their staffers recalled good-old days when the two of them had worked out deals on potentially controversial legislation, deals that the rest of the Finance Committee and the full Senate then endorsed. Wouldn't it be great if they could do it again? These two "old boys" of the Senate yearned for a repeat hurrah, but in Congress and the larger U.S. polity, the ground had shifted to open ideological crevasses under them.

Mere interpersonal agreements just cannot hold or shape visible policy outcomes any longer, at least on highly charged issues that split the parties. Grassley and other Republicans wanted to exchange their votes for a Finance Committee bill for firm commitments from Senator Baucus, President Obama, and Senate Majority Leader Reid that no further changes would be made in the Senate Finance bill as it was merged with another bill in the Senate and thereafter reconciled with whatever the House enacted. How could Senator Reid or the President ever make such a promise, committing hundreds of actors over several months? Were they going to tell all liberals in the Senate and the House, and in the entire Democratic Party just to buzz off, so they could do what Grassley wanted? Would progressive groups and activists allow Democrats in Congress just to sign on to a Republican-titled bill, no questions asked? Obviously, these were nonstarters. Equally fatal on the Republican side, Senator Grassley could never promise many Republican votes. His party leadership would not sign on. And even Grassley himself had ideological reservations—about the role of government in health reform—as well as practical worries. He was facing re-election and getting pressure from Republican and Tea Party activists in Iowa not to cooperate. Other Republicans he approached for votes would be pressured from the grass roots, too. Tea Party mobilization was happening even in supposedly moderate Maine, a fact that surely caught the attention of Senator Snowe.

The failure of interparty collaboration, including the inability of Baucus, Grassley, and the Gang of Six to seal a formal deal, was not the simple work of one villain, but resulted from mutual distrust in Congress, clashing electoral strategies, and omnipresent pressure from dueling activists who credibly threatened painful retribution. Nevertheless, at the level of substance rather than votes or public stands, the Gang of Six and other cross-the-aisle discussions substantially influenced reform. Indeed, the health reforms that Democrats ended up pushing forward on their own included new versions of ideas about regulated market competition articulated by Republicans all the way back to Richard Nixon, as well as, more recently, by Mitt Romney and the conservative Heritage Foundation. Paradoxical as it may be, Democrats in the U.S. polity as it is in the early twenty-first century have ended up engaging in what could have been bipartisan negotiations, working out, in their own ranks, what, in substance, are deals between old-fashioned moderate Republicans and various types of Democrats. But lest we think that Republicans substantively win even without cooperating on final votes, let's keep in mind that, after health legislation passed beyond the Senate Finance Committee, it moved back in certain ways toward the majority positions among Democrats. Unrelenting Republican refusal to join in bipartisan votes withdrew pressures for probusiness modifications and contributed to the formation of more liberal legislation in late 2009 and, especially, in 2010 than would have been possible if Republicans had carried through with their early negotiations.

WHAT WERE THEY ARGUING ABOUT?

So far, we have analyzed the politics of legislative sausage making without focusing systematically on the content of the new provisions that emerged amid the push and pull of partisan disputes, intra-Democratic Party deals, stakeholder bargains, popular pressures, and lost possibilities for a scintilla of official bipartisanship. We cannot get down to the substance by talking about a presidential plan that was accepted or modified. For all the talk about "ObamaCare" and the "Obama health care plan," there never was any such thing. At the outset of his presidency, as we have learned, Obama offered general principles for comprehensive reform—outlined in his first annual budget, in key speeches, and in the March 2009 White House Forum—and then handed the ball to Congress to carry down the field. The President's guiding goals for reform, echoed by other administration officials, were (1) widening access to health insurance and medical services; (2) regulating the private insurance industry to tame its mercenary habits; (3) raising new public revenues and trimming existing programs to help pay for expanded access; and (4) slowing down the overall rate of inflation in both private and public health care spending. As for hot-button social issues like abortion that could derail broad coalitions for reform, Obama always wanted Congress to downplay and defuse those longstanding fights.

Ideas about how to address each goal came from both sides of the partisan divide, but as we have learned, Democrats (plus two Independents) had to finalize provisions in the November House bill, for which they provided all but one of the 220 votes for passage, and in the Christmas Eve Senate bill, for which they provided all 60 votes. Here is an overview of what those bills forged in 2009 offered—sometimes through provisions endorsed by both chambers, and sometimes in contrasting provisions pushed forward by either the House or Senate.

Widening Access to Health Insurance and Services

Democrats and many Republicans agreed that health insurance should be much more extensively available, and polls consistently showed large majorities in favor of universal coverage. How to accomplish this, or something close, was the question. Washington Democrats started by accepting the existing employer system (for all the nonelderly except the poor), a system based on private insurance, employer-negotiated coverage, and the dominance of private medical care providers and suppliers. The White House and its Congressional allies were well aware that supermajorities (7 out of 10) Americans were dissatisfied with the coverage and insurance system overall, especially given its high and rising costs. But the Democratic leaders also knew that the public's evaluation of personal health coverage was positive or, at worst, mixed— only about a fifth were dissatisfied with their personal coverage or quality of care, while four out of ten were displeased with the costs they and their family faced. [61] Alert to the political peril of imposing changes that were disruptive to everyday Americans, DC Democrats routinely sought to soothe public anxiety by insisting that, as the President put it, "nothing" in emerging reforms "will require you or your employer to change the coverage or the doctor you have."[62] To the relief of many executives, Obama also declared that he had "no interest in putting insurance companies out of business."[63] To attempt any such thing, of course, would have aroused the anxiety and ire of hundreds of thousands of insurance company employees and may well have stirred up broader public unease.

Instead of blowing up the current system, the Democrats used a variety of mechanisms to expand its reach and improve its services and protections. One of the most important devices included in all House and Senate versions of reform called for the creation of "health insurance exchanges" or marketplaces where small businesses, individuals, and the uninsured seeking coverage could shop and compare prices and benefits among a variety of insurance plans. This concept was adopted by Republican Mitt Romney when he was Governor of Massachusetts, and was hailed by conservatives for introducing "the next stage in the evolution of a consumer-focused approach to health system change."[64] Exchanges equip consumers to choose among insurance plans by requiring insurers to offer packages of coverage that meet stipulated standards, while providing easy-to-understand information and call centers to help shoppers make choices based on cost and quality without fear that differences resulted from inadequate or fraudulent coverage. The Massachusetts model was used not only by Democrats but also in Congressional Republican proposals.

Although Democrats and Republicans largely agreed on health insurance exchanges, they disagreed on a key mechanism for eventually attaining near-universal insurance coverage—namely, a mandate requiring individuals to obtain insurance or else pay a fine. This is, in essence, like the requirement to purchase accident insurance before driving a car, so that if an accident occurs, people will have costs covered and the general public will not have to swallow the bill. Mandating most individuals to get insurance serves to pool the relatively small number of sick and medically expensive cases with the far larger number of healthy people, avoiding the problem known as "adverse selection" (which happens when insurance plans become lopsided with seriously ill people who are costly to treat). In the abstract, however, Americans dislike government mandates, and elected representatives worry about irritating voters by ordering them to do things. As Congress fashioned reform bills, exemptions were created for people who, even with federal subsidies, cannot afford insurance, as well as for people with religious objections. Even so, Democrats in Congress stuck with versions of the mandate, to kick in after 2014. Republicans in Congress, however, steadily backed away from this originally conservative idea, and, by the end of 2009, were vociferously denouncing it as a Democratic plot to violate American freedoms. No matter that the mandate had also been at the heart of Romney's health reform in Massachusetts and had previously been touted by some conservatives as a way to enforce personal responsibility and consumer-driven health care.

Requiring every American to purchase insurance on an exchange (unless covered already by their employers) would work only if people could afford the price. Reformers wanted to provide federally funded subsidies to make coverage affordable for lower- and lower-middle-income people. Democrats and the faction of Republicans who negotiated with reformers engaged in a lively debate about how large the subsidies needed to be to make the purchase of insurance feasible. Liberals wanted to help lower-middle-income families as well as low-income people, and were very worried about imposing a mandate to buy insurance without quite-generous help for people to meet the requirement. Republicans and more than a few Democrats cringed at the cost and pushed for more modest subsidies.

In addition to building new exchanges along with mandates and subsidies to generate additional insurance coverage for tens of millions of working-age Americans, policy makers discussed expansions to Medicare (the popular government program that now insures seniors) as well as improvements and expansions in Medicaid (a federally subsidized and state-administered government program that covers some poor people).

The Medicare debate focused on expanding the prescription drug benefit, which was added to the program under the presidency of George W. Bush, by reducing its "doughnut hole" in coverage. A way to pay for this would be to scale back or eliminate costly federal subsidies to private insurance companies running a special program within Medicare (called the "Medicare Advantage" program). Of course, private insurers did not want to lose Medicare Advantage subsidies that pad their profits, so they put up a lot of resistance; and Republicans proclaimed to older Americans that Medicare would be cut for all of them, even though three quarters of them were not in Medicare Advantage and were being offered a more generous drug benefit.

A lot of media attention was paid throughout 2009 to the arguments over Medicare but the eventual expansions in Medicaid were more important, though less reported upon. The policy debate over Medicaid for the very poor focused on two issues that, in the end, led to substantial expansions of state responsibilities—provoking the ire of certain governors. As of 2009, states determined how poor an individual had to be to qualify for its version of Medicaid, and some states covered only the extremely poor—as low as 11% of the federal poverty line in Alabama, which is equivalent to an income of only $2,425.50 a year for a family of four. Debates among Democrats in Washington focused on establishing a national minimal standard (rather than allowing each state to choose its floor) and setting eligibility above the federal poverty line (which was about $14,000 for individuals and a bit over $29,000 for a family of four in 2009). This would raise benefits for millions of poor Americans including many who worked full-time at minimum wage jobs. The second issue was whether to expand the types of people eligible for Medicaid from its core clientele (children, pregnant women, and the disabled) to include, as well, adults without dependent children. Again, a lot more poor people would get medical coverage. These debates revealed fissures among Democrats, too, because some states would have to spend much more than others in the future, depending on how many poor people were currently left aside in their Medicaid programs. Not just southern Republicans, but also some heartland Democrats—like Ben Nelson of Nebraska—were worried about the shares their states would have to pay in an expanded Medicaid program and bargained, with considerable success, for better terms for states that would have to do more in the future.

Reformers also worked out ways to widen access to specific medical services—long-term care for chronic illnesses; primary care; mental illness and substance abuse; and prevention and wellness programs. The political fireworks over health reform obscured attention to the serious discussions about such much-needed services among policy experts, community leaders, health care providers, and public-health advocates.

Could Private Insurers Make Money While Covering Everyone?

Before 2010, the private insurance business rested on decoding the traits of individuals (their health, gender, age, where they lived, and other factors) to determine who would be profitable to cover, and at what price. Steadily, private health insurers were moving away from the idea of pooling old and young, male and female, rich and poor, black and white, sick and healthy at average rates. For the young and healthy, individualized insurance was a boon, but it could be a nightmare if you were older or sick. Women who had paid premiums for years found their insurance policies terminated after they were diagnosed with breast cancer, or they suddenly had caps placed on how much insurance companies would reimburse them for their medical costs. The perverse fact was that the bottom line for private insurers depended on avoiding the sick.

Democrats and a number of Republicans broadly agreed that this dysfunctional health insurance business model had to be reined in, with companies nudged toward providing protection against (rather than avoiding) the cost of illnesses. Forbidding insurers from setting annual and lifetime caps on coverage or rescinding coverage after customers are diagnosed with costly illnesses are ideas that enjoyed broad bipartisan support.

But key disputes broke out between the parties and among Democrats of different ideological stripes over how deeply to regulate the insurance industry by, for instance, dictating the degree of different charges to be allowed for various age groups or requiring that insurance companies devote high percentages of their premiums to actual health care (as opposed to administrative expenses, profits, and executive bonuses). Liberal Democrats generally wanted to limit premium differentials and regulate more aggressively, and they had the most ability to shape insurance regulations in the majoritarian House.

Could Washington Pay for Promised Benefits?

Every policy maker who truly engaged in the 2009 debates over health reform knew that new programs and expanded insurance coverage or enhanced Medicare and Medicaid benefits would need to be paid for in some predictable way. Yet how to manage this divided the parties and disunited Democrats. Basically, Republicans would not agree to support any expanded health benefits that needed to be covered with new taxes—which meant that, as the year progressed, they were more and more clear that insurance coverage should not be expanded or improved significantly until after (as they put it) "health care costs are brought under control." Because this was to occur by means unspecified at some vague point in the future, Republicans opposed health reforms in large part because they did not want to raise new revenue for them.

But the issue of how to pay split Democrats, too. There were warring camps on several key issues: In the first place, many

Democrats in Congress wanted to counteract the unraveling of employer-sponsored health insurance in recent years by requiring businesses to pay a fee if they do not cover their employees and leave them to buy insurance with government subsidies on the new exchange. To go this route entailed arguments about which businesses should pay how much—and how generously small businesses might be treated (exempted from fines, given subsidies to insure employees, etc.). Many Senate Democrats were not willing to charge businesses as much as most House Democrats—and the bills produced by the two chambers reflected these differences.

A second financing dispute broke out about high-cost insurance plans offered by employers. There was significant agreement across party lines that these plans were unfair because their costly tax exemptions (which amounted to the federal government's third largest health care expenditure) were unavailable to many Americans and drove up medical costs by inviting excessive treatment by hiding the costs of such treatment. The 2008 Republican presidential candidate, John McCain, as well as several congressional Republican bills, proposed to remove entirely the tax exemption in favor of extending tax credits to all Americans to purchase coverage, whereas Democrats considered imposing a new tax on insurers who offered high-end plans to fund tax credits to help moderate-income Americans purchase insurance. Although Democrats did not seriously consider ending the tax exemptions as Republicans proposed, they disagreed among themselves about the so-called Cadillac tax on expensive plans that would, in essence, claw back part of the employer tax exemption. Obama and key Senate Democrats were convinced that this could be (as one White House aide explained) "your one lever on cost control in the private sector," but for many other Democrats, especially in the House and among Senators close to organized labor, any trimming of tax privileges for employer plans was a political loser, given determined union opposition.[65]

The third and perhaps most intense battle over financing erupted about whether to use general revenues from higher taxes on the rich to pay for health reform, as opposed to savings squeezed out of Medicare and private stakeholders. Republicans and a number of Senate Democrats (especially in the Finance Committee) opposed using taxes on the rich whereas many House and Senate Democrats wanted to tap general revenues, but they disagreed over the mechanism. Some liberal Democrats, especially in the House, favored using higher taxes on the most affluent Americans earning more than $1,000,000 per year (an idea the public approved in opinion polls), whereas others explored increases in Medicare taxes. The November 2009 House bill was considered especially liberal in large part because it used various tax-the-rich approaches to fund better benefits and subsidies for lower and middle-class Americans.

Can Expanded Access and Reduced Costs Really Go Together?

Throughout the recent health reform debates, President Obama pledged to "slow the growth of health care costs" and, in a point of high drama in his September national address, promised that he would "not sign a plan that adds one dime to our deficits" (marking a striking contrast with Clinton who used his veto threat against any legislation that did not achieve universal coverage).[66] Obama asked Congress to do what he and his White House green-eyeshade advisors believed was both possible and necessary: expand access to quality health insurance coverage, while "bending the curve" of rising health costs to reduce long-term projected costs in both the private and public parts of the system. The CBO "scores" were always anxiously awaited to see if new benefits were paid for and if costs were projected to be under control over one to two decades.

Although there is little question that Obama's White House believed expanded access and cost containment could go together, Republicans and fiscal watchdogs repeatedly raised questions about the willingness of Congress to take tough steps. It is easy to please constituents with better benefits, they reasoned, but when costs are reduced, that usually means that someone's profits or accustomed benefits are trimmed—which each politician is loathe to do, except to another politician's constituents or favorite business. In addition, Americans themselves never really believed the President's hopeful math or credited the CBO scores that projected long-term savings. People hear that the price for health reform approaches $1 trillion, and do not see that as cost saving. One reason conservative and Republican objections resonated with many in the general public was that people were skeptical about who would pay for new benefits.[67] The uninsured and underinsured might gain, people realized, but who would pay the higher taxes or insurance premiums to make that possible? Older Americans, above all, felt that they would pay through cuts in Medicare or greater difficulty seeing a doctor.[68]

In truth, designing a credible process for cost control was a challenge, because each significant proposal to rein in expenditures collided with an individual or organization that defined the particular kind of spending or a given tax break as necessary rather than flabby waste. Doctors and hospitals warned that reducing their reimbursement would have threatening consequences to patient care. Insurance companies and their representatives in Washington flagged the job losses from disrupting their firms. Medical device companies issued dire reports about lost innovation. Reduced spending on Medicare's Advantage program aroused opposition from its beneficiaries as well as from Republicans who suspended their long-running arguments against "entitlement spending" to make common cause with Advantage insurers and anxious older voters. The pattern was clear: consensus on the problem of rising costs, but intense disagreement about any and all possible solutions.

In the swirl of exhortations to control costs and protests against specific remedies, Democrats and some Republicans debated numerous approaches—including controversial ideas, such as malpractice reform to discourage lawsuits over medical errors and seeding new research on effective medical treatments. Both of these made it into bills as pilot experiments. In addition, lawmakers pondered ways to change modes of paying health care providers to encourage provider collaboration to further good patient outcomes, rather than reimbursing for each identifiable service provided—each discrete office visit, surgery, or day in a hospital bed. Pilot studies were authorized to experiment with extra payments to doctors and hospitals that deliver high quality care at lower cost, and bundling compensation to teams or integrated organizations that coordinate all services from hospitalization to the longer term care that many patients need after hospital treatment.

One of the most significant steps to contain costs, which might draw on the new demonstration projects and research, was the establishment of an independent commission to oversee Medicare payments and look for things to trim or streamline in the name of quality and cost efficiency. The key idea, pushed hard by fiscal watchdogs, is to insulate such decisions from the usual micromanagement by representatives in Congress influenced by lobbyists for medical providers and other industries that profit from Medicare. Sounds good in principal, but of course Congress people see this as "forfeit[ing]...our constitutional responsibility" and "hand[ing] off important authority to unelected officials."[69] In the 2009 bills, the House omitted this approach to cost containment, whereas the Christmas Eve Senate bill included it. This made sense, because House members are more sensitive to constituent pressures and anxious to retain their prerogative to decide on Medicare benefits and payments in each election cycle.

Additional, relatively noncontroversial provisions that might contain costs in the future involved speeding technological innovations. Few are happy with how the health system currently operates on a day-to-day basis. Doctors, hospitals, and patient complain about the hassle and cost of paperwork to justify reimbursements, and fiscal watchdogs turn red in the face over the waste and fraud. Lawmakers of all stripes agreed on encouraging the use of new information technologies to simplify everyday routines, pool information on patients for teams of providers coordinating care, and probe for signs of waste or fraud.

Dodging Old and New Controversies to Get the Bills Through

When the House and Senate voted on their final bills in November and December, each chamber crystallized its overall solution to combining access and cost controls. The House version made concessions to fiscally conservative "Blue Dog Democrats," yet it also contained relatively liberal approaches to taxing the rich, requiring businesses with fifty employees or more to contribute to health care coverage, and offering new Medicare benefits and generous subsidies to enable low- and middle-income Americans to buy insurance. The House included a watered-down "public option" and, significantly, a unified national insurance exchange. The Senate's Christmas Eve bill included provisions friendlier to business and health-economy stakeholders; and it opened the door to further concessions down the road by charging the fifty states, rather than the federal government, with administering health insurance exchanges. The Senate also excused larger as well as smaller businesses from ironclad contributions to universal health coverage. At the same time, the Senate took cost control ideas more seriously, including two provisions refused by the House: the Medicare Payment Commission and a tax on Cadillac health plans.

Last-minute fights over hot-button social issues could have divided Democrats enough to derail votes for reform bills in each chamber. An old issue—whether the federal government will in any way pay for abortion services—almost undid the

House Democratic coalition, until, at the last minute, Speaker Pelosi allowed conservative Democrat Bart Stupak of Michigan and his allies to schedule an additional vote on draconian abortion restrictions on private plans to be offered in new insurance exchanges. Prochoice Democrats resented this deal, but accepted it to let reform squeak through (as it did 220 votes to 215). A newer social issue—the place of undocumented immigrants in the future reformed health system—reared its head in both House and Senate. Latino and liberal lawmakers wanted immigrants, including undocumented people, to be able to purchase coverage with their own money in new exchanges, but more conservative Democrats, egged on by Republicans, wanted ironclad provisions to deny "illegals" any benefits from the reformed health system, even if they paid for them. These matters had to be fudged, or compromised toward the more conservative positions, to keep comprehensive reform bills moving.

Fitfully, with many near breakdowns, the bills did keep moving. Speaker Pelosi and Majority Leader Reid both delivered what President Obama had requested early in the year. Before the end of 2009, each leader corralled enough votes from their caucuses to enact legislation—in slightly different versions due to the different rules and makeup of the House and Senate—that promised to expand access to more than 30 million currently uninsured Americans and at the same time control costs and improve medical care delivery. Both leaders, and their Democratic majorities, pushed the boulder of comprehensive health reform almost to the top of the mountain— and they hoped to reconcile the two bills and push that heavy rock all the way over the top immediately after the New Year.

3

HOW THE SCOTT BROWN UPSET STRENGTHENED HEALTH REFORM

Conventional wisdom in U.S. politics can turn on a dime—and turn again. It happens all the time, yet the winter of 2010 will go down in history for especially dizzying gyrations. First health care reform was a nearly done deal; the boring business of backroom negotiations in DC was all that stood in the way of its enactment. As people trickled back from a too-short recess, union leaders pressed the White House to drop charges on expensive health plans. At the same time, staff members in Congress haggled to reconcile the House version of reform, which taxed the rich to offer more generous benefits to regular Americans, with the Senate version that offered tougher cost controls and was a bit more to the liking of business and the well-to-do. Irritating as these differences were, and tricky to resolve, insiders had no doubt that, very soon, a compromise version of historic health reform would go back to the House and Senate for final votes and proceed to the President's desk for a signing ceremony before the 2010 State of the Union Address.

Then, suddenly, health reform was pronounced dead—victim of a sudden heart attack on a gray, wintry special election day in Massachusetts. On Tuesday, January 19, Scott Brown, an obscure GOP state senator and populist darling of the Tea Party, shocked the political world by upending an apparently sure-thing Democratic nominee to win, of all things, the Senate seat held for the previous forty-seven years by deceased liberal health reformer Ted Kennedy. The political gods seemed to have played an especially ironic trick, as Brown openly campaigned to become the forty-first vote to sustain a Senate filibuster to kill "ObamaCare." After his election, he rushed to Washington to do just that.

"David vs. Goliath," the Brown campaign was dubbed by the *Boston Herald* (a Murdoch tabloid not given to subtlety), which explained how the "Upstart's Surge Threatens Leader of the Free World's Agenda."[1] From the evening of January 19, conservatives and Republicans could barely contain their glee. "ObamaCare went into the emergency room in Massachusetts and didn't make it out alive.... The health care bill...is dead with not the slightest prospect of resurrection," declared Fred Barnes in a middle-of-the-night posting on the Web site of the über-conservative *Weekly Standard,* which also enumerated the collateral political benefits conservatives were about to realize. Barnes confidently predicted a much weakened President Obama and a hobbled House Speaker Pelosi, who was deluding herself if she still thought reform could pass, along with demoralized Democrats likely to retire rather than face punishing races for Congress in the fall, and a "new king of Capitol Hill," Senate Minority Leader Mitch McConnell, whose "skill in keeping 40 Republicans united against Democratic health reform was masterful."[2] For weeks, it looked as if Barnes was right.

But flash forward two months later to the first day of spring. On Sunday, March 21, a beaming Nancy Pelosi presided as the House passed comprehensive health reform by 219 votes to 212 (a larger margin than the House vote back in November 2009), and two days later, a triumphant President Obama, surrounded by cheering Democrats, signed into law the Patient Protection and Affordable Care Act of 2010 (or Affordable Care Act for short). As amended in a prenegotiated way, comprehensive health reform became in some ways bolder and more liberal and therefore even less appealing to Republicans than before Scott Brown won. Back in Massachusetts, the *Boston Herald* again captured the essence of the moment. "Gleeful Dems, shaken Repubs ask: Where Is He Now?" was the headline, juxtaposed to a picture of a troubled-looking Scott Brown with a label plastered across his forehead that read "Best if used by March 21, 2010." "Republicans feeling blue as Scott Brown win backfires," explained the full story, which quoted Democratic leaders crowing that "'Scott Brown's election actually delivered health-care reform,'" because it "inspired...procedural means to bypass GOP efforts to derail the bill."[3]

Health care reform thus went from healthy, to stricken, to resurrected and bolder during the first three months of 2010. How did this happen?

WHY DID A SINGLE ELECTION SEND DC INTO PANIC?

Just one seat was at stake on January 19, 2010. After the Brown upset, as well as before, Democrats remained overwhelmingly in the majority in both House and Senate. Why was the election such a big deal? Why did it paralyze health reformers and DC Democrats for many weeks in the depth of winter? The answer lies in a toxic combination of surprise, distrust among Democrats, and fear of electoral contagion.

How Could This Happen in Kennedy's Home State?

First, there was the sheer surprise factor. Only about ten days before the Massachusetts contest did it begin to dawn on Democrats that they could lose this election. Massachusetts is the most liberal state in the nation, and before the special Senate election there were *exactly zero* Republicans in its delegation in Congress and in its statewide offices—a sure-fire formula for complacency during a time of nationwide voter disenchantment. After the Democratic Senate nominee, Attorney General Martha Coakley, coasted to an easy win in a special fall primary, she assumed she had the Senate seat in the bag, took time off over the holidays, and then visited DC to confer with bigwigs. But she should have been scrambling. At the end of 2009, people in Massachusetts, as throughout the nation, were worried about a poor economy with vanishing jobs and sluggish commerce, and irritated that all the DC politicians seemed to be talking about were unsavory deals to complete a huge, expensive, incomprehensible health reform (one that seemed less essential to Massachusetts, because the state already has pretty much the same system, created under former Republican Governor Mitt Romney with support from, among many others, State Senator Scott Brown!). Along with virtually every other state government grappling with desperate budget trade-offs during the recession, the Democrat-led Massachusetts state government was also unpopular.

Although he is much wealthier than Coakley, Republican hopeful Brown drove around Massachusetts in a pickup truck, speaking out against "the Democrat establishment" in Boston and DC. He was regularly featured on the popular Sports Radio Station, WEEI, especially the 6–10 A.M. "Dennis and Callahan Show" that mixes sports commentary with Republican talking points—and mocks liberals as "out of touch."[4] Coakley gave the radio jocks plenty to work with; she kicked off days of ridicule by misidentifying revered former Red Sox pitcher Curt Schilling as a New York Yankee fan, and also publicly pooh-poohed the idea of standing in front of Fenway Park to greet voters. Brown, meanwhile, made good mileage declaring he would go to DC to block "big government" corruption like the Cornhusker Kickback. He suddenly had plenty of television and radio ads. Once it became clear that a Republican actually might win in Massachusetts, the Tea Party mobilized to hold signs and run rallies, even as national conservative advocacy groups, the Chamber of Commerce, and other financial and economic interests spent millions to support the endgame.[5] By the time the Democratic National Committee, leading unions, and Organizing for America (Obama's campaign apparatus) began to pour Democratic resources into the race, it was already too late. Even the President's visit the Sunday before the election proved futile. Many Massachusetts voters who had supported Obama in 2008 (and still liked him) stayed home, while droves of blue-collar workers voted for Brown.[6]

The Brown upset thus happened in a relatively unionized state, where workers have a long history of voting for Democrats. An election-night poll called the election "'a working class revolt'" because Democrats were "'not successfully addressing workers' economic concerns.'"[7] Driven by economic and political disaffection, Massachusetts voters elected a new Senator who ran on his opposition to national health reform modeled on their state's plan, even though a *Washington Post* poll found 8 out of 10 voters supported the Commonwealth's new health system.[8] Of course, part of the explanation for defection by Massachusetts workers may have been rooted in worries they were hearing from union leaders about pending health care bills in Congress. National union leaders had spent early January castigating health reform for possibly including a "tax on the middle class," their label for the tax on high-end employer benefits included in the Christmas Eve Senate bill. Even though the White House agreed to scale back this tax, days before the special election, few Massachusetts workers had heard this, so they remained worried. In effect, many Massachusetts union members fixated on national union criticisms of pending DC health reform bills, and bucked their state leadership on the Senate vote as such. Union households supported Brown by 49% versus 46% for Coakley, and thus played a critical role in giving the Republicans their forty-first vote to stymie all union priorities in Congress, including national health reform![9]

"Panicking Is What Politicians Do When They Lose Elections"[10]

Democrats' shocked surprise at the Massachusetts upset soon led to mutual distrust and fear. To be sure, efforts outside Congress to prevent bad news from killing the almost-completed health reform started even before the polls closed in Massachusetts. Liberal pundits and bloggers, led by such influential commentators as Josh Marshall at *Talking Points Memo* and Steve Benen at *The Washington Monthly,* started days before the election to urge Congressional Democrats to remain quiet and calm if Brown should win. Commentators also explored ways to get health reform passed without sixty votes in the Senate Democratic caucus.[11] By mid-January, the White House and leaders in Congress had agreed upon final adjustments to the 2009 bills, so maybe the compromised legislation could be rushed through both House and Senate in the ten days or so it would take Brown's victory to be legally certified.[12] Or perhaps adjustments between the House and Senate bills from 2009 could be included in a special "reconciliation" bill with fixes to taxes and spending, which would be eligible under existing rules to pass the Senate with a majority (rather than the sixty-vote supermajority). And then there was the easiest option: just have the House "pass the damn bill" (as Steve Benen repeatedly urged), that is, accept the 2009 Senate bill with no changes, declare victory, and leave all kinds of improvements in benefits and shifts in taxes desired by the House majority for another day.[13] The 2009 House and Senate bills agreed on 85% or more of all provisions that would go into comprehensive reform, so why was that not good enough, asked many commentators.[14]

Hours before Coakley conceded to Brown on January 19, the President pushed this course in a quickly convened Oval Office confab with disheartened House Speaker Pelosi and Senate Leader Reid.[15] Just getting it done would save his place in history without a lot more Congressional sausage making. Pelosi was renowned for always rounding up votes for the President's priorities, but she told her colleagues straight out, the "Senate bill is a non-starter," that she could never assemble a House majority for accepting it unmodified.[16] Just nine-and-a-half months before all her members would have to face the electorate, she would be asking fiscal moderates to swallow the hated Cornhusker Kickback, and trying to get progressives to accept benefit and tax provisions not to their liking (including the tax on employer health plans opposed by unions). For every House member, the next election loomed, and Representatives were not about to walk the plank by accepting unpopular measures to coddle the slow-moving Senate. "I can't sell that to my members," Pelosi said.[17]

Truth be told, the usual interbranch tensions were already at a high point before the Scott Brown election threatened to make Congressional gridlock unbreakable. As a change-oriented President asked for many new laws throughout 2009, the House responded by passing dozens of significant bills—many of which had only gone on to die in the Senate, deadlocked by supermajority rules and Republican filibusters.[18] Pelosi heard constant grumbles that her House people were voting for things that could be used in negative attack ads, yet were not actually carried into laws with accomplishments they could tout to their constituents. Brown or no Brown, she could not ask for any more unpopular votes, certainly not in deference to the resented Senate—and she told Obama and Reid just that.

The evening ended without any clear Presidential or DC Democratic plan to move ahead on health reform—and, of course, blogger pleas for Democrats in Congress to stay calm fell on deaf ears. When the President did not immediately propose a way forward, the Congressional Democrats, badly frightened, ran around like chickens with their heads cut off. If this kind of electoral loss could happen in the liberal state of Massachusetts, even with the President making a special appeal for the Democratic candidate, what would happen to many of them facing tough re-election fights in November? "The absence of a clear statement from the White House," seasoned Washington reporter Elizabeth Drew explained, "led panicked Democrats on Capitol Hill to make contradictory and often incoherent statements."[19] Each Congressional Democrat went his or her own way, and in many cases gave voice to anxiety or timidity on camera. As if his state had not already done enough damage, influential and loquacious Massachusetts House member Barney Frank grumbled that health reform was dead.[20] Centrist Senator Evan Bayh of Indiana argued that the Brown election should be a lesson to Democrats to change tactics, and Senator Jim Webb of Virginia took mere hours to declare that there would be no more votes until after Scott Brown was seated, thus ruling out any possibility of a quick enactment of the compromises already on the table.[21]

Learning that there was no painless way forward in Congress, the White House also went into a period of uncertainty—and issued vague or conflicting statements about health reform for days and weeks after the Bay State upset. "Obama Retreats on Health: President Tries to Salvage Overhaul's 'Core Elements' amid Capitol Hill Chaos," trumpeted a day-after *Wall Street Journal* headline that foretold what would keep coming.[22] From some of the morning-after public statements, it sounded as if Obama was considering once again Rahm Emanuel's idea of scaling back health reform, perhaps into halfway measures or symbolic steps.[23] "Kiddie care" was reportedly the derisive response from Nancy Pelosi, who would continue to press the White House to orchestrate true cooperation between House and Senate.[24] Grappling with unpleasant political facts post-Brown, Obama realized that half-way measures were nearly impossible, because the various parts of comprehensive reform are so interdependent: insurance regulations don't work unless everyone has coverage, and everyone cannot afford coverage unless government helps. Still, he continued to oscillate, giving some speeches signaling determination, and others hinting at retreat.[25] In his much-parsed January 27 State of the Union Address, the President remained elusive. He lectured Democrats not to "run for the hills" and "walk away from reform.... when we are so close." But he also said nothing specific to explain how Congress should proceed and on what basis. Congressional Democrats became openly angry with the White House, blaming it for not sorting things out and leading the way with a substantive plan and procedures to get it done. "There's no level of trust between the Senate and the House or the White House and everyone else," a longtime Democratic insider told Elizabeth Drew.[26] Congressional frustration with Obama's lack of clear direction sparked new U.S. Senator Al Franken to lash into Obama's political lieutenant, David Axelrod, in a closed door session with Democratic Senators in early February: "Goddamn it, what's the deal here? ... You're talking platitudes, and.... [w]e're getting the crap kicked out of us!"[27]

As paralysis and interbranch distrust deepened, little happened beyond ritual declarations that health reform would not be dropped. This is how big undertakings die in Washington, DC. Politicians always say they are not abandoning the important priority, but they stop doing things to move it along and allow even almost-completed legislation just to fade away. As of February, this looked like the fate of the health reform effort that had eaten up an entire year in Washington.

Anger and Black Humor from the Democratic Base

Watching the DC disarray, dismay and anger spread among health reform advocates and the Democratic Party base. How could the largest Democratic majorities in decades walk away from the almost-completed century-long quest for comprehensive health reform? Black humor broke out. The *Village Voice* headlined an article "Scott Brown Wins Mass. Race, Giving GOP 41–59 Majority in the Senate."[28] On the *Daily Show,* Jon Stewart "explained" why the Republicans were now in charge.[29] Likewise, a wicked football cartoon by Toles made the rounds, showing team "Dems" in a quarterback-less huddle. Down by five points, preparing for the last play of the game on fourth down at the one inch line, the Dems were debating whether to punt or kick a field goal!

Indeed, as the weeks of winter unfolded, Democratic voters and donors showed increasing signs of disgust, their

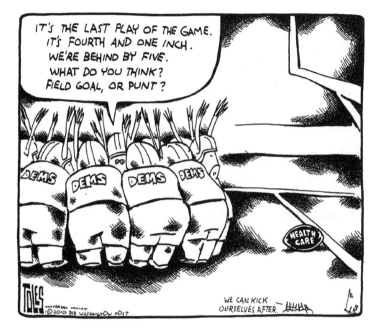

mood perfectly captured in the Toles cartoon. Core Democratic supporters felt that Obama and the Democrats in DC should get things done now or risk having their base voters stay home in the coming fall Congressional elections, and maybe in 2012, too. If that happened, the Republican dream of repeating their party's 1994 rout could come true, with energized Republicans heading to the polls, while many Democrats stayed home in discouragement. After all, both the House and Senate had *already voted* for health care bills that opponents had, to some degree, successfully demonized in public opinion. The material for more anti-Democrat campaign ads was already there, so things could not be any worse—and might improve, if Democrats in Washington actually passed final legislation and had something to show for their efforts. This message got conveyed to Washington, not only by poll responses from Democratic voters, but also by party loyalists who threatened to withhold checks or even run challengers against Democrats who failed to support health care reform.[30]

HOW WAS HEALTH REFORM REVIVED?

It took Democrats in Washington weeks to calm down and clearly grasp the tough choices and possibilities available to them. But at last they came out of their funk and began to look for ways to finish reform. In due course the Brown victory in Massachusetts spurred Democrats to cut out the incessant posturing and cooperate to finish comprehensive health reform—in a bolder and better form. A wide array of national interest groups who, in the end, wanted something rather than nothing to pass, also quit maneuvering over details and pushed, all together, to help Obama and the Democrats in Congress get it done. Everyone from unions and the AARP, to the American Medical Association and the *National Catholic Reporter* got on board in the final weeks. The lone wolf efforts of some progressives to revive the public option fell flat as other progressives and Democrats focused on pushing the ball across the goal line.

Things began to turn in earnest when progressive organizations led by the Center for American Progress and Health Care for America Now, working in tandem with the White House, were able to focus national media attention in February on plans for a huge 39% rate hike announced by Anthem Blue Cross in California, a subsidiary of the private insurance mega-corporation WellPoint.[31] President Obama, Health and Human Services Secretary Kathleen Sebelius, and Congressional Democrats—all seized on this and additional pending rate hikes to "reignite[] the health reform push," as *American Medical News* put it.[32] Suddenly, the threat of unregulated insurance to small businesses and individuals became vivid again. Even Fox News—firmly opposed to pending health reform legislation—admonished WellPoint for (in the words of

Business Channel host Stuart Varney) handing "the politicians red meat at a time when health care is being discussed...."[33]

The President Steps Up

During February, the White House also concluded that the Massachusetts vote, and public opinion more generally, exemplified anger at the messy DC process and end-stage deal making in 2009, more than clear opposition to specific parts of reform (like regulation of insurance abuses or expansion of benefits) that continued to be popular.[34] Republicans, in contrast, banked on global poll responses that showed a majority of Americans opposed to the "proposed changes in the health-care system being debated in Congress."[35] Believing the public to be with them, Republicans called for the year of effort to be scrapped, for Congress to just "start over" from scratch. But of course they did not really mean start over. There was no chance that Republican leaders would abandon their apparently successful strategy of just saying no to President Obama's major legislative priorities. After Brown's election, that approach looked like a winner heading into the November midterm elections—so the Massachusetts outcome absolutely ensured that health reform would get no Republican support in Congress. Why would even moderate GOP Maine Senators Snowe or Collins support Democratic bills in the wake of a victory by the Republican candidate in the Senate election held just to their south?

Deciding yet again to advance rather than retreat in the face of political headwinds, President Obama finally took ownership of a specific plan for comprehensive reform, and moved to draw the spotlight off maneuvers in Congress that had proved so off-putting to voters. White House confidence in Obama's ability to control the public agenda rose following the State of the Union Address, when he accepted an invitation to make remarks—and take any and all questions—at a Republican House retreat. The President's staff arranged to have this remarkable encounter televised. Surrounded by lions in their den, Obama did a masterful job of rebutting specific claims put forward by House conservatives, who rose one after another to try to trip him up. It made for a riveting show that Obama clearly dominated.[36] Soon after, the White House decided that the next big step to "get health reform done" would be a televised "bipartisan summit," to be convened at Blair House across the street from the White House, on Thursday, February 25. Congressional Republican leaders were not thrilled and understandably griped that this was just a gimmick to pave the way for a last-ditch attempt to pass health reform. But how could they refuse to attend without looking like cowards or obstructionists?

Three days before the Blair House Summit, the President publicly issued "his own" comprehensive plan—essentially a clearly written summary of the agreed provisions that House and Senate negotiators had already arrived at.[37] He invited Republicans to have their own plans "costed out" by the CBO, urging them to propose specific alternative ways to cover more than 30 million Americans without insurance, and also to control rising health care costs. Making a big show of saying he was open to "better ideas" for reaching these popular goals, Obama knew full well that Republicans would not offer many viable suggestions. The purpose was to let the American public see the contrast between a Presidential plan to get things done, and Republican nay-saying.

The Blair House Summit came and went with no breakthrough to bipartisan comity. No surprise there. After seven hours of speeches, posturing, and an occasional snippet of true dialogue, with Obama present throughout to display his mastery of health care issues, little changed overall. At the end of the day, Obama made a show of asking Democrats in Congress to add a few more Republican ideas to their legislative write-ups, but everyone knew that make-or-break had come. It was up to the Democrats to proceed, or else fold. They would get no Republican votes. What the public theater directed by

Obama did achieve, however, was to convince Democrats in the House and Senate that he was taking visible responsibility for finishing health reform. Congress would not be alone. Furthermore, their party's president was laying down the gauntlet *to them:* He was staking his presidency on health reform, and making Democrats in Congress responsible, should they not heed the call, for causing a Democratic President to falter just a year into his first term. Obama was playing for keeps.

Congressional Democrats Get Their Act Together

Public choreography by the White House in late February also gave Pelosi and Reid time to finalize interchamber compromises in quiet negotiations, where they persuaded their colleagues to go along with a majority-vote, filibuster-avoiding procedure endorsed by the White House, giving reform "an up or down vote" in Congress. In essence, a two-step process would be used to get around the forty-one-vote Republican filibuster bloc in the Senate. The House would pass the 2009 Christmas Eve Senate bill, along with a so-called sidecar bill that would enact various changes in taxes and spending agreed upon in advance with Senate Democrats. This sidecar bill would then be passed by simple majority in the Senate, using the established procedure known as "reconciliation," by which fiscal bills can avoid filibusters. In the past, Republicans had repeatedly used this approach to pass tax cuts benefiting wealthy Americans[38]—so their outcries about process would be less convincing than they might otherwise be.

The genius of this plan was that it allowed Congress to build on all that had been accomplished in 2009. The difficulty of the plan was that it required House Democrats to trust Senate Democrats to carry through with the sidecar vote. Pelosi had to persuade her House caucus that the Senate would not just pocket their vote for the original Senate bill and then bog down, as the Senate typically does. She stressed that the

President backed the full plan, and required Senate Majority Leader Reid to present, in public, a letter signed by substantially more than fifty Senate Democrats promising to carry through with a vote on the sidecar bill, no matter what (a commitment they eventually kept, even in the face of having to cast embarrassing votes against all kinds of mischief amendments offered by Republicans).[39]

Of course, all of this still looked like more sausage making in press reports. Obama was doing his best to make the endgame for health reform a transparent, public, televised process, to take visible presidential ownership of reform and describe the specific provisions to the American people. Still, health reform remained huge and complicated—and the public remained fearful.

Substantively, there were ironic ways in which the endgame allowed the eventual Affordable Care Act to become bolder, more liberal, and certainly less weighed down with special side deals. With fifty-one rather than sixty votes now the hurdle in the Senate, Ben Nelson and a number of other Democrats who traded votes for special deals back in December lost their leverage. The Cornhusker Kickback was removed in the sidecar. And even though the Senate bill provided the overall framework, the sidecar allowed the House to reduce and delay the "Cadillac tax" on generous employee health plans that the unions and their allies opposed. To find alternative sources of revenue to pay for expanded health insurance for low- and middle-income Americans, the House persuaded the Senate to accept higher taxes on health-care industries, and higher fees for wealthy Medicare beneficiaries (including a new tax on income from Wall Street and other financial investments). The Senate and the White House, however, pushed the House to accept a cost-monitoring commission for Medicare. Many House members disliked this, but it was a provision important to getting good scores from the Congressional Budget Office. Final CBO scores projected long-term savings and documented that the Senate bill plus sidecar would not only pay for health reform but actually cut the federal deficit. This was crucial, because dozens of Blue Dog moderate and conservative Democrats in the House were skittish about voting for a nearly trillion-dollar reform package, and Pelosi and the President persuaded many of them by stressing that health reform would help to control the ballooning federal budget deficit.[40]

Another step to help with those CBO scores was a nifty compromise involving previously passed House legislation on aid for college students.[41] The House wanted to cut subsidies that allowed banks to reap a profit on loans to college students made with no risk to the banks (because the government would cover defaults); the federal government would instead make direct loans to college students at a lower cost. This would save the taxpayer more than $60 billion over the next decade, which the House originally planned to use exclusively for enhanced Pell Grants for lower-income college students and other forms of aid to higher education. This legislation, like many other 2009 House bills, had stalled in the Senate, because Ben Nelson and a few other Senators would not vote for it, leaving it shy of 60 votes to break the usual Republican filibuster. But after Brown arrived and the Democrats came up with the reconciliation sidecar to get around the filibuster, the opportunity arose to add in the educational reforms because the votes of Nelson and other conservative Democrats were no longer necessary. This made House liberals happy; they could go home to their districts and brag about making college more affordable for low- and middle-income families. At the same time, Blue Dogs were pleased, when about half the savings from the student-aid reforms were rerouted within the sidecar bill to help defray the cost of health care reform and contribute to reducing the budget deficit. Everyone in the House Democratic caucus got something, and the CBO scores improved.

Even with compromises working out and a fragile trust building between House and Senate Democrats, the final two weeks before the March 21 vote brought high drama. Pelosi remained just short of the majority she needed, as she and

President Obama held dozens of one-on-one meetings to per-suade holdouts.[42] Obama delayed a trip abroad and invited House members, mostly fiscally worried Blue Dogs, to a jaw-boning session in the Oval Office. Even for members of Congress, meeting the President in the Oval Office is a special honor and most fell into line after talking with the President, creating a steady stream of announcements of favorable votes. On the other side of the spectrum, when the President took a trip to Ohio to sell health reform in a town meeting, he made sure that left-wing holdout Representative Dennis Kucinich was on Air Force One, so he could overcome his doubts about supporting a bill that lacked the "public option" desired by liberals. The next day, Kucinich backed off from his long-term opposition to the kind of reform embodied in the Affordable Care Act, and he actually began to reach out to other Democrats in Congress to build the majority.[43]

A few last minute deals had to be worked out, including revised provisions to satisfy Representatives from the Midwest and Pacific Northwest that their states would be fairly treated in Medicare reimbursement formulas.[44] Yet final interchamber discussions were complicated by the fact that only some things could be adjusted from provisions in the 2009 Senate bill. Given the procedural difficulties post-Brown, the Senate bill had to be voted by the House as the centerpiece of the comprehensive reform, and only the fiscal aspects—money matters having to do with taxes and subsidies—could be changed in the sidecar bill. Anything having to do with administrative structures or regulations had to remain just as it was in the 2009 Senate bill, because such matters were not, by rule, suitable for the recon-ciliation sidecar. The Senate parliamentarian would rule them out of order.

On one critical matter, the House just had to back down. The November 2009 House bill called for a unified, national exchange for health insurance plans—and this would have made the implementation of reform and its operation a more streamlined, efficient process. But the Senate had voted in

December for exchanges to be run through the fifty states (or through compacts among the states), and because of the Republican filibuster, this provision had to remain frozen in place. The same was true for the regulations voted by the Senate about abortion—a fact that created great difficulties in completing the House majority on Sunday, March 21.

In the countdown to the House vote, conservative Democratic Representative Bart Stupak of Michigan, supported by somewhere around half a dozen allies (the exact number was shifting and uncertain), was still refusing to accept the Senate bill language on abortion.[45] Stupak and his group wanted additional assurances that abortion services could never be paid for by any subsidies offered to Americans purchasing health insurance on the new exchanges. Were they using the abortion issue to scuttle health reform entirely? It was not clear, and everything was going down to the wire with Pelosi possibly just short of her House majority. On Sunday afternoon, a few hours before the scheduled vote, the President promised to issue a specific Executive Order right after the House vote to reinforce the bans on public abortion funding already in the pending legislation. This step, combined with courageous public support from leaders of more than 60,000 Catholic nuns and other consecrated religious women, as well as from hospitals represented in the Catholic Health Association, finally allowed enough prolife Democrats to vote for health reform—against the urgings of the Catholic Bishops who, to the end, remained allied with the Republicans in opposition to the reform legislation.[46]

At last, comprehensive health reform had the votes to pass— with the House vote at 11:37 P.M. that Sunday night. Following shortly after its approval of the Senate bill, the House passed the sidecar legislation, which then headed to the Senate. Various details between the chambers were settled a week later, but for all intents and purposes, March 21 was the key vote: Comprehensive health reform would become law as soon as the President signed the Affordable Care Act.

Passions boiled over at the end. As Representative Stupak provided articulate support for the health care reform on the House floor, he was denounced as a "baby killer," not just by Tea Party protesters in the streets and the House gallery, but also by a colleague, Republican Representative Randy Neugebauer of Texas.[47] When the final legislation passed with solely Democratic votes, liberals and moderates who had yearned for health reform were both relieved and delighted, but conservative dismay continued. Inside and beyond Washington, DC, conservatives were frustrated that they had almost, but not quite, created a Waterloo for a change-oriented President they strongly resented and feared. With Brown's surprise victory in Massachusetts, Republicans had been so sure they could stop "ObamaCare" that the ultimate passage became a still-more bitter pill for them. House Republican leader John Boehner loudly denounced the legislation from the well of the House as "Armageddon" that will "ruin our country."[48] After Affordable Care passed, there were denunciations and calls for repeal. Congressional Democrats endured racial and homophobic epithets from protesters the day of the House decision, and a number were threatened with outright violence as they returned home on recess right after the historic votes.[49]

A New Course for America

Political differences would not go away, as conservatives "reloaded" to continue battling for repeal. What is more, the enactment of comprehensive health reform did not automatically change reality on the ground. That would come only after months and years of implementation of an intricately fashioned new framework for regulating and financing health care. Yet as the winter of 2010 turned to spring, one thing was sure. The huge boulder that was enabling legislation for comprehensive health reform had, finally, been pushed over the top of the mountain in a U.S. polity that, by design, makes big reforms very difficult to achieve. The Patient Protection and Affordable Care Act—urged to completion so doggedly by President Obama, Speaker Pelosi, and Majority Leader Reid—went into the books as one of the most important pieces of social legislation since Social Security, Civil Rights, and Medicare. It promised to put the United States on a new path—toward affordable health care for all Americans.

4

WHAT DID THEY DELIVER? THE PROMISE OF AFFORDABLE CARE

Americans have reacted to the passage of the Affordable Care Act with sustained ambivalence, with those disapproving of "ObamaCare" exceeding those who applaud it overall. People were put off by months of partisan battles, judicial challenges, and the rocky start in 2013 for the health insurance exchanges where consumers can select health plans and receive subsidies to help pay for them. But when pollsters ask Americans about specific provisions in the law, supersized majorities of 60% to 80% support core features such as new rules for insurance companies and subsidies and tax credits to make health coverage affordable for almost all American families and businesses. This schizophrenic response—ambivalence about "ObamaCare" as a whole but support for its key features—happens because most Americans do not yet have a firm grasp on what is in the new reforms or what they mean for their families and the country.[1]

Doubts and confusion are understandable. The new law is a complex blueprint requiring enormous changes that were bound to produce hiccups and uncertainties. An uncertain economy leaves many people worried about costs and taxes, and opponents have worked overtime to fan doubts and spread frightening falsehoods (such as the lie that "death panels" will cut off medical care for the elderly). After decades of experience with laws fashioned in DC that turned out to help banks, corporations, and the superrich while middle Americans are left struggling, why shouldn't people worry that it will happen all over again with this big health plan?

This chapter traces the aims of the Affordable Care Act enacted in 2010 and checks in five years later to see how its performance matches up. We lay out what reform accomplishes for Americans in different life situations and probe its impact on the economy and the national budget in which we all have a stake. Bumps in the road were to be expected—and have occurred—but here's the bottom line if you have been distracted by the political attacks or the incessant carping in the media: The Affordable Care Act as judged by careful independent analysts has delivered on expanding access to tens of millions of Americans and controlling budgetary costs for U.S. health care overall.

Much will depend on whether the provisions put on paper in 2009 and 2010 can be fully carried through as intended amid swirling interest groups and contending partisans. We deal with the results of legal challenges and the ongoing politics of implementation in chapter 5. But first, let's get straight what the Affordable Care Act says and what difference it is making for various groups of Americans, for the overall functioning of the U.S. economy, and for the national budget.

WHO BENEFITS FROM HEALTH REFORM?

A simple, honest question needs to be asked and answered: How are most Americans affected by health reform? Olympic-quality rhetorical gymnastics are performed to avoid a straight-forward and objective answer, but here it is: *The winners of health reform are the vast majority of Americans.* As the provisions are effectively implemented, senior citizens, the sick, and average Americans—including many families in the upper middle class—are now receiving wider and easier access to health insurance benefits protected from trickery by the insurance industry. The number of working-age Americans and their children who have to go without basic health insurance is on track to decline by a remarkable 26 million people. This comes from the nonpartisan Congressional Budget Office (CBO), which projects that coverage will ultimately be extended to 92% of all Americans and legal immigrant residents (up from 83% in 2010).[2] About a third of the remaining uninsured will be undocumented or illegal immigrants, who are not eligible for coverage under the reform law.

Taking into account all parts of reform—including regulations to make insurance more secure for those who already have it—Americans of modest and middling means reap most of the benefits, while additional costs are picked up by the most economically advantaged. The bill for health reform will be paid by multibillion dollar corporations in the health insurance industry, by pharmaceutical producers, and by medical-care providers, as well as by slightly higher taxes on very rich families (individuals whose yearly incomes exceed $200,000, or married couples earning more than $250,000). The tax dollars raised from those at the top are mostly to be used for subsidies to reduce the premiums paid by millions of middle-income Americans, and also to help people working for low wages who have been unable to afford private insurance in the past. The bottom line for the vast majority of Americans is *more benefits, greater security, less cost.*

Americans who enjoyed good health insurance in the past through employment or other sources are seeing better protections from arbitrary decisions by private insurers than would be the case without reform. As in the past, insurance remains mostly private; and so will medical treatment. Health care reform brings needed care to the previously uninsured and allows most people to keep seeing the same doctors and receiving treatment for themselves and loved ones at the same or comparable clinics and hospitals. As President Obama explained, this "isn't radical reform. But it is major reform."[3]

The more detailed realities of America's emerging new health system are best described by zeroing in on how important groups are affected: seniors who are naturally nervous about the Medicare benefits they already count on; young adults trying to get started in a down economy; middle Americans juggling bills to make ends meet in a turbulent job market; economically strapped families who are struggling to get ahead; and also the most affluent among us—folks who saw their piece of the economic pie dramatically expand during the past four decades and wonder what will happen now. Here are the plan's implications for each group.

Retirees on Medicare Get Many Benefits

Nearly 46 million Americans rely on Medicare to pay for their medical services. For the 70 percent of Medicare recipients who are in the mainline Medicare program, the reform means nothing but good things. It offers a smorgasbord of new and improved benefits:

- *Sharp reductions in the cost of pharmaceutical medications.* Medicare beneficiaries received in 2010 a $250 rebate for drug costs that fall into the "doughnut hole" between $2,700 and $6,154—a gap where they have had no assistance to pay bills in the past. By the end of this decade, the new reform will pay for 75% of prescription drug costs, and the prices charged by pharmaceutical companies will be sharply reduced for Medicare recipients.
- *Expansion of primary care.* Reflecting a growing realization of the country's shifting medical care needs, the reform increases Medicare's payments to doctors in family medicine and general internal medicine and offered them a 10% bonus from 2011 to 2015. Everyone on Medicare is now able to develop a personal wellness plan each year that identifies what risks they need to reduce and what tests they should receive that year. The reform encourages coordinated service for older Americans, not just cooperation by doctors, but also nurses

trained to catch problems before they spiral into medical emergencies, and routine help from social workers who can help senior citizens with the challenges of everyday life. Recommended preventive services are now provided free to Medicare recipients. These common-sense improvements introduce new ways to reduce costs and, at the same time, provide higher quality care to older Americans—solving problems early to help seniors avoid unnecessary hospital visits.

- *Protection against the all-too-common abuse of seniors by family members and care providers.* Borrowing from laws to prevent child abuse, the new reform encourages the development of protective services for the elderly, including background checks for those seeking employment in nursing homes and other long-term care facilities, and improved oversight in medical treatment facilities.

Thirty percent of Medicare recipients as of 2013 were enrolled in "Medicare Advantage" programs, which doled out taxpayer subsidies to private insurance companies to offer coverage. Those enrolled in Medicare Advantage enjoy the benefits just discussed, but what about their own plans? To help pay for the cost of new drug benefits for all Medicare beneficiaries, the reform law reduces taxpayer subsidies to private insurance companies offering Medicare Advantage plans, starting in 2012. Doomsday predictions that insurers would drop seniors or jack up premiums and co-payments have proved to be unfounded. Medicare Advantage plans have remained affordable for seniors who want them, and enrollment has increased since Affordable Care was passed.[4]

Young Adults Just Starting Work Get a Leg Up

America's youth are given new protections as they volunteer or start their first meaningful jobs—good news at a time when they face special challenges breaking into the labor market.

- Regardless of whether sons and daughters go to college, parents can keep their young-adult offspring on the family insurance plans until the age of 26.
- Also, for the first time, young adults can qualify for Medicaid if their annual income is low ($14,444 or less in 2010). Many times, wages are low at first, so this can ease young adults toward a place in their careers where they either get insurance through employers or can afford to buy it themselves (bolstered by extra help from public subsidies until their incomes reach a threshold where they can cover premiums on their own). As a result of the Supreme Court decision to give states the option of accepting or rejecting expansions of Medicaid, 30 states have adopted the new expansion with more on the way. Nonetheless, in every state, hospitals rely on Medicaid to pay for the care of the uninsured, and under the Affordable Care Act the federal government will pay all of the cost for the first three years, with states eventually contributing merely a nickel toward each dollar of federal funding.[5] In the end, we predict all states will go along with the planned expansions. (By way of comparison, it took nearly two decades for all states to adopt the original Medicaid program after it was passed in 1965.)

Middle-Income Americans Will Enjoy Affordable Insurance and Improved Care

Health reform also benefits millions of middle-class Americans, people who work for a living and need affordable and secure insurance coverage from employers or individually purchased plans. The central idea of the reform is to make decent health insurance affordable for all Americans and U.S. businesses—and then require everyone to participate responsibly in the system to avoid shifting costs onto their neighbors.

Affordable Insurance. The new system uses about half of its $1 trillion in new spending to help individuals and small businesses with fewer than 50 employees afford health insurance.[6] Millions are receiving subsidies to help pay for premiums in the four out of five U.S. households earning less than $95,400 a year (as calculated in 2014), including people who now, or at some future point, need to buy insurance without participating in a big employer-run plan. This is freeing millions of people to take care of a family member or pursue economic advantages wherever they may be found—without worrying if a new job carries insurance. More and more Americans have similar chances to get good, affordable coverage no matter where they work.

Specifically, families of four with annual incomes up to four times the federal poverty line ($95,400 in 2014) are entitled to subsidies to pay for insurance premiums. Small businesses with fewer than 25 employees and average wages less than $50,000 a year also receive tax credits to cover 50% of their contributions to the premiums of their employees. In a novel departure, nonprofit enterprises are also able to use these tax credits. The new system builds in a backstop to make sure that premiums remain within reach: low-income Americans do not have to pay any more than 2% of their income, and this cap slowly rises to 9.5% for those earning up to four times the federal poverty level.

Special interests trying to scare Americans have claimed that insurance premiums will go up as reform is implemented (as if they have not been going up sharply all along!). What scaremongers deliberately do not mention are the subsidies and limits we have just highlighted. For Americans receiving insurance on the government exchanges, new health care subsidies produced lower net costs for millions of Americans and moderated the costs for others.

As the Affordable Care Act made its way through Congress, the CBO estimated that after accounting for subsidies the average cost of buying insurance in the individual market would fall nearly 60% by 2016, and the cost for those in small groups, such as employees of small businesses that buy coverage, would decline by around 10%. CBO changed its estimate four years after reform was enacted—they reported that the average premium was 15 percent less than their initial estimate. Private insurance companies did raise premiums for plans purchased at work but only modestly—3 percent during 2014.[7]

Fairer Insurance Markets. In 2009, before health reform passed, about a third of nonelderly Americans had no health insurance from employers, and instead purchased coverage in the most expensive and least secure part of the insurance market—the so-called individual and small group markets.[8] The new health reform helps such Americans in many ways. First and foremost, reform allows people without employer insurance to participate in new insurance marketplaces known as "exchanges," where they enjoy the same choices and advantages previously limited to employees of large businesses. The new law equips individuals and, eventually, small businesses (with 100 employees or fewer) to shop among competing sets of standardized private insurance packages (from the "Platinum Plan" and other plans to the "catastrophic option" for people under age 30 that pays just for very high expenses that might occur after a serious accident or illness). Individuals and businesses shopping on the new exchanges have considerable freedom to find the option that is affordable for them and offers the coverage they prefer. Good old-fashioned competition appears to be motivating insurers to design the best coverage plans for the lowest price.

There are commonsense rules of the road on the exchanges, to avoid the worst possibilities we all know from the past about the dog-eat-dog world of private insurance. The reform sets new rules for minimum services, and limits on how much insured people can be charged out of pocket. It also requires private health insurance to cover basic preventive checkups for no extra charge. New rules of the road for insurance exchanges also stop insurers from using misleading and obscure "fine print" to confuse customers. Exchanges prepare easy-to-understand descriptions of coverage options, and they establish a call center, facilitate enrollment, and simplify citizens' application for subsidies to help pay for insurance plans. More than a dozen states made solid progress in establishing the new exchanges, and the Federal government is now smoothly operating exchanges individually tailored to serve citizens in 34 states.

The makeover of private insurance markets has been surprisingly smooth. The prices of premiums for plans offered on the exchanges have been more moderate than the CBO initially projected, and in most states more insurers are offering plans than originally expected. Good prices and growing participation by insurance companies and nonprofit plans are indicators that the new health insurance markets are working.

Opponents of reform have exaggerated glitches along the way as Affordable Care transitions America to a new, fairer system. Insurance companies marked the arrival of new rules of the road in fall 2013 by sending out cancellation notices to people who had previously subscribed to shabby plans, and critics of ObamaCare declared that five to six million Americans were losing insurance. Back in the real world of objective data, some people did lose access to older plans and had to pay higher premiums in return for more generous policies. But about two-thirds of Americans who lost policies became eligible for tax credits to help them afford new, more secure coverage.[9]

Better Care. In addition to expanding access to health insurance, all Americans are gaining improved access to vitally important new services as the nation's health care system begins a potentially momentous shift toward prevention and wellness, a transition expected to lower costs and make life better. New payment formulas and rules in the Affordable Care Act encourage the provision of essential medical services through family medicine, general internal medicine, pediatric care, and community clinics. The new system eliminates copayments or deductibles for immunizations, checkups, and screenings for a range of potential illnesses from cancer to depression. American families are projected to save hundreds of dollars each year, and many of us are starting to enjoy bonuses that could amount to thousands of dollars in return for responding when our employers ask us to consult with a "health coach" or fill out a risk assessment to help pinpoint preventive services. A representative of large businesses praises these new steps as "transformative" in helping to move U.S. medicine from a "model that was based on treating illness and injury, to a model that's focused on improving an individual's health and identifying risk factors.[10]

In an important breakthrough, Affordable Care brings a new hope for Americans suffering from mental illness and substance abuse. For the first time, insurers must cover treatment for these crippling illnesses as they do for other diseases, and medical providers are encouraged to integrate treatment for mental and addiction disorders into ongoing primary care.

One of the likely challenges in the future will be handling increased demand for care by Americans who, in the past, were unable to afford it. New funding and incentives are geared to expanding the pool of front-line primary care doctors and nurses to meet the demand for essential care. Unlike most other affluent democracies, the United States has historically had far more specialists than general practitioners. With little public fanfare, the Affordable Care Act is preparing to respond to the new demand for medical care by reconfiguring the balance in favor of first-line care givers.

Getting Everyone into the System. With insurance plans made affordable for all, every American is required to use a combination of subsidies, employer support, or personal income to obtain an acceptable health insurance plan, or else pay a financial penalty of up to $2,085 for a family ($695 for individuals).

Exceptions exist, including for people who have a religious objection or can demonstrate unusual financial hardship when premiums are more than 8% of their income. For almost everyone, this system is proving practical, because insurance plans are widely available and affordable in one way or another.

Nevertheless, enemies of reform have demonized the "individual mandate" rule that everyone have health coverage. They know how easy it is to scare Americans into thinking they might be affected by bureaucratic rules or asked to pay "taxes." But the claim that the mandate is a vast "middle class tax" is preposterous. Non-partisan experts estimate that the vast majority of Americans—98% to 99%—have not been affected by the mandate rule at all.[11] Only people who can afford insurance but do not have it from employers or public plans are at risk.

If so few are directly affected, why bother with the mandate at all? The logic here is the same as for car insurance. All drivers have to buy basic coverage, so that if an accident occurs, the costs are not just shifted to other citizens. Similarly, everyone must have health coverage, so that people cannot just appear at the emergency room and foist the costs onto the hospital or their neighbors who pay insurance premiums and taxes. The idea originated with conservatives, who saw it as a simple instance of personal responsibility. The 2012 Republican presidential candidate, Mitt Romney, justified the mandate that way when, as Governor of Massachusetts, he sponsored the same approach to health reform as the one now extended to the whole country in the Affordable Care Act. The best way to keep premiums affordable for everyone is to require everyone to pitch in, while helping all citizens and businesses find affordable choices for health coverage.

Before moving on from middle-class Americans, let's pause for a moment to highlight how clearly this new Affordable Care system builds on the established routines we have long been accustomed to in the United States. As in the past, the new system continues to depend on private insurers and private doctors, nurses, and health care providers—all of whom continue to purchase the valuable products of private manufacturers of medications and medical devices, businesses that continue to make good profits and to employ millions of people. There is no government takeover here, because the centerpiece of the reformed system is a competitive marketplace of private insurers seeking customers, looking to attract more citizens and business clients based on the quality of the health plans they offer at a good price. Indeed, many of the core components of this system have been advocated by conservative economists and Republican policy makers impressed by the benefits of competitive markets. Affordable Care uses conservative means to pursue progressive ends.

For all the hype about the supposed disruptions, the Affordable Care Act builds on the best features of our existing system to make them available to all Americans.

Help for the Most Vulnerable

Along with seniors, young adults, and middle-income Americans, the most economically vulnerable people in our country are also winners in the reformed health care system. Before 2010, three-quarters of the 50 million Americans without regular health insurance were our neighbors—folks caught short by an illness but not covered at work and without wages high enough to pay the high costs of insurance or care on their own. Consider three types of Americans who had been uninsured before 2010 and who are now being covered as the new program is implemented:

- A 35-year-old single mom who is employed at a small business with no benefits, earning $40,000 a year, whose son suffers from diabetes.
- A 60-year-old single woman, who left the workforce to care for her own mother and dropped her own coverage after the premiums became unaffordable.

- A 56-year-old man and his 52-year-old wife who do not have children and left the workforce because of bipolar disorder, alcoholism, and a raft of resulting medical issues, and have to get by with $21,000 annually from retirement programs and a modest inheritance from their deceased parents.

All of these Americans, who had lacked or lost insurance, can now receive it. The system of exchanges and subsidies helps the single mom purchase private insurance, and it bars private insurance companies from refusing coverage based on her son's diabetes.

The older single woman and married couple can escape from the morass of medical bills they cannot pay. First, private insurers are barred from omitting them and hiking up their premiums. Our imagined cases (and many other Americans) can also benefit from government incentives to employers to continue to offer insurance to early retirees.

The middle-aged couple grappling with bipolar disorder and alcoholism is now eligible for a range of services that might help them re-enter the workforce. In a historic breakthrough that has received little attention amidst the political food fight, America's new health system recognizes mental illness and substance abuse as illnesses and mandates insurance to treat them.

People like those we just described can also benefit from *substantial expansions of Medicaid*, the longtime federally subsidized and state-administered program for those with low income. More Americans will be eligible, as Medicaid is redesigned to grow (along with its parallel program for children) to cover 16 million more enrollees. Although it may take longer in some states than others, the new Medicaid program will widen eligibility to include adults without children (rather than primarily limiting it to children and pregnant women), and raises the income level for eligibility to a nationally consistent 138% of the federal poverty line. In plain English, that means eligibility for families of four making up to $32,900 in 2014, and for individuals making up to $16,104. Medicaid expansion will cost 45% of what the new health reform is projected to cost overall, so it is a big deal.

Yet another important breakthrough has received less attention than it should. Community health clinics in urban and rural areas are being built, refurbished, and expanded to treat about 4 million more people—nearly a 25% increase since President Obama was inaugurated. Six out of 10 of the new patients are from ethnic and racial minorities and about a third lack health insurance and are kids. The Affordable Care Act is investing $11 billion in expansion of a system that Republicans and Democrats alike have worked to create over the past half century.

The Affluent Benefit, Too—and Pay Much of the Bill

As we have spelled out, the newly reformed U.S. health care system provides, on balance, a good deal for the vast majority of Americans. At the very top of the economic ladder, though, the payoff for families making more than $250,000 a year is mixed. They share in general improvements in insurance, and, of course, many wealthier Americans place a high value on a better health care system for all their neighbors, as well as for themselves. They want their children to grow up in a healthier America, where teachers and policemen and clerks can enjoy health security, too. Still, the rich are asked to pay a bit more to make this better system possible.

On the plus side of the ledger for privileged folks, richer families benefit along with all other Americans from new restrictions on insurance companies that prohibit caps on coverage and egregious abuses such as finding a pretext to drop beneficiaries when they get sick. This has happened even to rich people in the past, although, in truth, the rich have often been able to purchase premier coverage out of reach for most Americans. And they are less likely to get pushed around by insurance companies, because they may be able to get on the phone and call the CEO!

On the cost side for the very-well-to-do, Affordable Care does what substantial majorities of Americans have repeatedly told pollsters they would like to see—tax the rich who have reaped the largest share of the gains over the past four decades to support benefits for the majority.[12]

Let's get straight exactly what this means for people at different levels of income, because the airways are filled with a steady stream of overheated claims. Affordable Care includes somewhat higher taxes for the small number of married couples with incomes greater than $250,000 a year (or $200,000 for individuals). Such well-off Americans face two significant changes in their Medicare taxes: they will pay 2.35% of their wages (up from 1.45%), and also a new tax of 3.8% on investment income (from the stock market, real estate, and other forms of high finance that are out of reach of all but a few Americans). Millionaire families are hit the hardest, paying more than three quarters of the new taxes—on average about $46,000 more a year by 2013. Affluent but not superrich families earning $200,000 to $500,000 a year pay modest additional taxes each year—about $560 on average, all told. Although scare tactics make it sound like all Americans face higher taxes, the truth is that the new revenue—to provide health insurance for 25 million Americans and lower the burden on millions more—is being paid by the most affluent 3% of households. In America's New Gilded Age of fabulous riches at the top, 90 percent of the new taxes are paid by the richest 1 percent at a cost that amounts to pennies to them—2 percent of their after-tax income.[13] Affordable Care's funding represents the most progressive tax reform in several generations.

Let's also be blunt about who is not subject to new taxes. Americans making middle-class incomes—people earning less than several hundred thousand dollars a year—who sign up or receive coverage are not directly hit by large new tax bills. The nonpartisan and widely respected Tax Policy Center reports that 97% of Americans (all but the very wealthiest top 3%) will be free from owing any additional Medicare taxes—the ACA's largest new tax on Americans.[14]

WILL HEALTH REFORM HELP OR HURT THE ECONOMY?

Health reform impacts the economy in ways that help everyday Americans, while producing an overall boost to job growth. People are now able to build careers and businesses secure in the knowledge that they can get affordable insurance for their families. Employers have to navigate new rules—and larger employers may pay new fees. But all employers benefit from more fluid job markets, healthier workers, and reduced costs— especially for employers who have already been providing health care coverage for their employees. The new responsibilities of large and small businesses were delayed to facilitate a smooth transition and are now in the process of being implemented.

As for businesses in the U.S. economy's vast health care sector, they are winners, on balance, enjoying more customers and opportunities for growth and profits. "Wall Street Welcomes New Health Prescription," proclaimed a banner headline in the business section of a leading metropolitan newspaper right after Congress voted on Affordable Care. Traders in health industry stocks know how to penetrate the partisan and ideological fog to see the economic bottom line.

Lest we think that only Wall Street wins, so will the Main Street economy. Without comprehensive health reform, perhaps a quarter of U.S. workers were locked into their jobs— afraid to pursue new openings out of concern to hold on to health benefits, or choosing a less than optimal job because it has health benefits and an otherwise more attractive job does not. "Job lock" is certainly bad for Americans trying to get ahead. And it is bad for the whole economy, too, because a mobile workforce is more dynamic, efficient, and entrepreneurial.[15] Assured health coverage also helps employees avoid lateness and absence from work, because many people come down with preventable illnesses or have to scramble to deal with emergencies better handled through routine care. For example, in the existing patchwork U.S. health care, prior to the full implementation of reforms, children of uninsured, low-income workers are often taken to emergency rooms for asthmatic attacks that could have been prevented through routine physician care. A mother or father loses work time, and the entire episode increases the country's health care bill because hospital treatment is far more expensive than routine medical care. Affordable Care includes many provisions to make routine care more available and affordable for all Americans.

Affordable Care supports families in many ways—most obviously, by making regular care available to children and parents. It also helps some of us with an aging parent or a sick member of our family to choose to take time off from work to give them loving attention.

Sixty percent of Americans receive insurance through employers who help pick up the cost of premiums, and Affordable Care includes provisions to reinforce the security and lower the cost of employer health plans with which people are happy. Large employers are slated to get help to pay health premiums for their retirees.

In addition, the new health reform requires larger employers who have not previously offered coverage to start pitching in—either to offer coverage or pay fees to the public to offset taxpayer subsidies for their uninsured employees. This will bring new costs to businesses with 50 or more employees that have not previously offered coverage or that offer coverage that is unaffordable or skimpy. The common-sense idea is to prevent free-riding by businesses that used to ask everyone else to cover their employees when they showed up in emergency rooms without insurance or—as would happen in the new system—when taxpayers help their workers with tax credits to buy affordable plans on the new health insurance exchanges. Having some businesses refuse to insure their workers creates an unfair marketplace, penalizing other employers who sacrifice part of their profits to meet their responsibilities to offer employee health coverage. Nor would it be fair to have taxpayers make up the difference. Provisions in the new law seek to correct or prevent unfair imbalances, and the entire national economy does better if the playing field is relatively level for businesses as well as workers.

A common criticism of health reform is that, in this or that instance, higher taxes or fees on business could depress job growth. What happens if an enterprise with 48 employees, just below the threshold at which federal requirements kick in, contemplates hiring two more workers? In truth, it does happen from time to time that a medium-sized business without insurance for its employees decides to put off hiring to avoid governmental charges levied on businesses with fifty or more employees. We may well see businesses gaming the new system in other ways. But most businesses most of the time do not plan their workforces around tiny shifts in taxes or fees; they take into account market opportunities and the costs and the uncertainties of making changes. And any government program is going to have thresholds. Affordable Care is actually generous in exempting most small businesses from rules and taxes, providing small and medium-sized responsible employers with generous tax breaks to insure employees, and agreeing to temporary delays of the law's original timeline. The greater fluidity and fairness this reform create for businesses overall outweighs the minor glitches and effects from those who game the system.

The doom and gloom portrayal of the impact of health reform on jobs is wrong according to non-partisan analysis.[16] Indeed, Affordable Care may create jobs in the health insurance market, health education, and medical care to meet new demand—one of the country's fastest growing industries. It may also give a boost to the economy by enabling consumers to spend some of the money they once devoted to insurance and care.

Charges that Affordable Care is responsible for job "loss" are partisan spin—not supported by expert analysis. The CBO reported in 2014 that reform did coincide with a "decline in the amount of labor that workers choose to supply," but the agency clearly stated that this drop was not the result of "an increase in unemployment." Workers simply have more choices now. No longer locked into jobs for health coverage, working people now have the option to leave their jobs to go back to school, launch a small business enterprise, stay at home with children, or care for a parent. All those are good things.[17]

In short, sky-is-falling warnings about the impact of health reform on businesses amount to little more than a lopsided political talking point. In truth, new realities are taking shape in the economy: enterprises are hiring new workers to meet fresh opportunities in health-related sectors; and employers are operating on a more level playing field, with all required to contribute to health care and all poised to benefit from employees with more secure access to one of life's necessities.

CAN THE NATION AFFORD ALL OF THIS?

Talking about all the good things Affordable Care delivers for patients in need of health care and for employers and workers who need to pay for good care can leave all of us wondering: yes, lots of goodies, but can America afford them? The estimated price tag for health reform is about $1 trillion during its first decade. That's a big figure. Many Americans are understandably leery about how this bill is being covered, and by whom. Watching the country's debt balloon after tax cuts mostly for the wealthy, two wars, eye-popping rescues for Wall Street and Big Auto, and a slew of domestic programs created or expanded during the first decade of the twenty-first century, many Americans of all partisan persuasions are wondering if it all costs too much. Could health care reform be the straw that breaks the camel's back?

According to the design of Affordable Care, the mammoth bill is to be paid by the affluent, well-to-do businesses, and established medical providers. Just over half the bill for health reform is covered, as we detailed earlier in this chapter, by taxes and fees that fall on the wealthiest Americans and on businesses (including health care giants and employers that have been free-riders in the past). The remainder of the revenue to defray costs in health reform comes from trimming what the federal government and nation were previously slated to pay over many years to health care industries and providers. Significantly trimmed subsidies to private insurance companies involved in Medicare are a substantial source of savings. "Bending the curve" is the term for this—and it reflects the fact that even if only slight reductions can be made now in the rate of price increases charged by physicians, hospitals, and health care companies of all sorts, such slight reductions can nevertheless add up to big savings over time. The authoritative and nonpartisan CBO projects that the law's combination of increased revenue from taxes on the affluent, plus cost restraints, will more than cover the price tag for health reform. Better, the CBO projects that future federal expenditures on health care will come down from previously assumed levels enough to *reduce the federal government budget deficit by about $140 billion during the first ten years of the new program*. CBO projects further improvement in the bottom line for deficit reduction during the second decade of Affordable Care. In short, Affordable Care as enacted is a deficit-reducer, not a budget buster.

Affordable Care's original design was not a pipe-dream; the budgetary bottom line over its first five years has turned out *better* than anticipated. The growth of health care spending ranged from 16 percent per year in the 1980s to 9 percent range in the early twenty-first century; it dropped to 3 to 4 percent after Affordable Care—the slowest rate in 50 years. The always cautious CBO made a bold pronouncement in April 2014: the precipitous decline in health costs reduced the budget deficit below its earlier estimate by $5 billion in 2014 and, during the next decade by $104 billion; a few months later, it reported a budget reduction of "more than $150 billion."[18]

In the stormy battles over health reform, comparatively little press coverage was devoted to the extensive discussions among policy analysts and Democratic and Republican policy makers about hitting the brakes on rising health care costs. Understandably, many Americans have concluded that Washington was merely engaged in handing out more goodies, expanding benefits, and was not paying any attention to the equally important job of applying the tough love of saying "no" or "not so much." The truth is that the Affordable Care Act includes an elaborate four-pronged strategy to reduce spending in certain areas, and also slow the overall rate of growth in public and private health care expenditures. These strategies are showing encouraging signs of making a difference.[19] The Act further stipulates that cost savings should be made in ways that primarily fall on the shoulders of the already economically advantaged. Let's look in more detail at the framework for cost control built into Affordable Care.

Reset Business Models for Insurers and Pharmaceutical Manufacturers

The first prong of cost control has been to reset the business models of the health care industry. In the first place, insurance companies, drug and medical-device manufactures, and health care providers are all required to reduce their charges or pay new taxes—and we are already seeing that such rules are moderating price increases. Beyond that, the new health insurance exchanges, and the arrangements they include to equip individuals and small businesses to compare coverage and costs in health plans, are starting to reorganize the private health insurance marketplace and create new incentives for delivering quality care at lower prices. The exchanges are inducing insurance companies to compete for profits, not by avoiding the sick, but by lowering premiums and their own administrative costs. Exchanges may also prod insurers to drive better bargains with doctors and hospitals.

Giant private health insurance corporations are not all that popular with the American people, and they have enjoyed near-monopoly profits in the past. Therefore, in designing ways to pay for Affordable Care, Congress and the White House hit the insurers particularly hard. Insurers with Medicare Advantage plans used to get a lot of gravy from the federal budget, because they got subsidies well above their per-patient costs. This is slated for cuts, $156 billion over ten years from insurers.[20] Insurance companies have already been compelled to spend 80–85% of their premiums on the true costs of medical care, rather than on administrative bloat or CEO salaries; those that failed to meet this new standard have already been required to rebate nearly $2 billion to policyholders. In addition, insurers are now barred from excluding customers with preexisting medical conditions, rescinding coverage of subscribers who become severely ill, or imposing caps on how much they will pay over a year or a lifetime for a given subscriber. The news is not all bad for insurance executives, though, because Affordable Care enables many more people and businesses to purchase coverage and Wall Street has rewarded the industry well.

Discourage Overuse of Medical Care

Influential economists have long argued that health care spending is rising too fast because generous insurance shields customers from the true costs of medical care. These economists insisted that Americans who are insured against all costs have a "why not?" attitude when it comes to demanding expensive medical tests or treatments even if they offer little value.

The new law imposes an excise tax on insurers for expensive employer-sponsored health insurance plans—those that are annually priced over $10,200 for individuals or $27,500 for family coverage beginning in 2018. This new "Cadillac tax" is expected both to raise revenue and to introduce a new "is it worth it?" attitude when it comes to requesting nonessential care. The Affordable Care Act will prod individuals and businesses to replace Cadillac plans with new plans that force patients to put some skin in the game by requiring them to pay higher deductibles and other costs. Some economists believe that this excise tax will have considerable impact on private sector health expenditures because it will discourage demand for unnecessary and costly care.[21] Even if this does not happen, the Cadillac tax may help to reduce costs to the government. Many of the beneficiaries of the most generous insurance plans already enjoy well-paid jobs—they are among the most affluent Americans who are slated to help pay for reform overall. Other Americans who have very generous employer plans are part of the small section of the workforce that is covered by powerful unions; they may end up paying a fraction more of their income for health care after 2018, but the impact will be slight.

Apart from the top end, Affordable Care will introduce a pervasive awareness of costs among the insured. For the first time, the W-2 forms that we get each year before filing our taxes now list our employer's contributions toward premiums. These contributions will not be taxed but they will reveal one of the great secrets of health care—how much we pay and how much we are giving up in wages to have health insurance. This delivers on the pleas of economists for transparency about costs. If they are right, it may fuel the cost awareness that we bring to buying airline tickets to choosing health insurance. This is one of many provisions aimed at cost control that has received little public attention.

Reduce (Still Growing) Expenditures on Medicare

Projected to grow sharply in future years, Medicare's payments to doctors, hospitals, and other medical providers were in the crosshairs of health reformers because of their magnitude ($504 billion was spent on Medicare in 2009, including 27% going to hospitals and 18% to doctors). Medicare also matters because the program's reimbursement rules tend to set standards for private insurers and payers as well. If, over time, the public pays a bit less than it otherwise might for Medicare, this will make a large difference in the overall rate of increase in health care costs in the future. Trimming payments to hospitals and to medical specialty physicians today will lower their base pay tomorrow, which over time will add up to tens of billions of savings.

The striking feature of the cost trims for Medicare built into Affordable Care is that they are primarily aimed at lowering reimbursements for comparatively well-to-do medical professionals and established medical facilities—leaving benefits the same for seniors and others who depend on the program. A lot of public fuss has been made—and will keep being made—about how bad Medicare cuts will supposedly be for senior citizens in general or doctors in general. Much of the brouhaha is misplaced, because primary-care doctors are not the target, and the vast majority of Medicare beneficiaries see only new benefits from Affordable Care, not cuts or new charges. Furthermore, as Americans live longer, Medicare will pay enough to cover retirees. At issue is the rate of increase in costs and the efficiency of payments, not sufficiency of coverage.

One of the most significant steps to rein in Medicare costs in the future was the establishment of a 15-member independent commission to find the best treatments at the best cost, thus restraining overall national health expenditures.[22] The idea is to have medical experts consider what works well and what should be paid to hospitals and doctors—and have the Commission's proposals automatically take effect unless Congressional majorities vote otherwise and are able to override a veto if the president supports the Commission. Lobbyists for the health care sector do not like that they will have less leverage through Congress—and a lot of Congressional people did not like it either. This provision got into the final legislation only because President Obama insisted. Furthermore, the legislation explicitly protects everyday

Americans, because the Commission is prohibited from changing Medicare's benefits, eligibility, or out-of-pocket charges. If the Commission exercises its powers, it may well restrain costs even more effectively than CBO estimated. The Commission also has the potential to extend its impact from Medicare to a still broader restraint of private health care costs. The bottom line remains, however, that any cost savings are targeted to come from reductions in already high salaries and the increased profits expected by relatively well-to-do providers. Providers will get more money—just not quite as much more—and regular Medicare subscribers should see no substantive difference.

Happily, the rate of increase in Medicare spending has slowed to levels not seen for several decades.[23] If this continues, Affordable Care will have contributed significantly to "bending the cost curve," putting all of U.S. health care on a more sustainable course.

Reconfigure Medical Practice

It will come as no surprise that dollars drive the medical industry. How medical providers are paid impacts who is treated, how well they are treated, and how much care is provided and when. The current practice is often to pay doctors and hospitals for each identifiable test, treatment, and office visit. Naturally, they respond by boosting the sheer volume of tests, treatments, and visits to increase their income. Patients are not usually knowledgeable or assured enough to say no to more tests, visits, and so forth. Especially when facing an emergency or a grave condition, most patients readily agree with the recommendations of doctors. Even the most ethical doctors experience intense pressures to increase the volume of (insured) care, and this is even more true for hospitals with budget shortfalls. Research suggests that perhaps a third of medical care lacks scientific justification.[24]

Little press attention or public discussion focused on the intrepid effort of experts and a select, bipartisan group of lawmakers to instigate a gradual transformation in how medical care is delivered within the new Affordable Care framework. The goal is to improve the quality of care and drive down costs by avoiding unnecessary tests and treatments. To this end, a number of Affordable Care provisions encourage new ways of paying medical providers to focus less on quantity and more on the quality of overall patient outcomes. Also included are support for experiments with payment systems focused on teamwork among medical providers and support for research on which procedures work best at the lowest cost. Funding was also provided to set up projects to explore alternatives to the current medical malpractice system that relies on lawsuits and court judgments, addressing an intense concern of many doctors.

Affordable Care has generated plenty of talk about "coordinated" and "performance-based" care, but major transformations in medical delivery have yet to emerge. The CBO has refused to score most of the experiments and new incentives as certain to deliver cost savings. It is hard to tell what will work—and the medical professions and organized providers often resist changes in long-accustomed practices. Nevertheless, the determination and purpose is clear—reorganize how doctors and hospitals operate in order to help pay for expanding care to tens of millions of underserved Americans. The steps to reconfigure medical care reflect the collective wisdom of a generation or more of health economists and health policy experts. Although many provisions may not work as intended, Affordable Care invites an extraordinary period of innovation and experimentation and the greatest opportunity in decades to deliver better health care at lower cost in future years.

THE BOTTOM LINE: BOTH BENEFITS AND COST-CONTROLS MAY WORK

Taking into account all four of the prongs of cost-control we have just summarized, it is clear that measures to keep the nation solvent are a prominent part of Affordable Care. The 2010 health reform challenges the simplistic tendency to equate cost with quality, a notion that has been misused by many U.S. providers to justify charges that far surpass what their well-paid counterparts collect for comparable quality care in Canada and western Europe. Health policy experts and many thoughtful observers of all political stripes have concluded that our nation can achieve higher quality health care at lower cost. Affordable Care establishes many of the new rules of the game necessary to realize this goal.

Critics complain that the new law does not require sudden, immediate cuts in health expenditures, but instead establishes new regulations, charges, and commissions to impose and spread the pain down the road. These are reasonable criticisms but miss what was done and why. In truth, health reformers developed a shrewd political strategy to induce weighty economic stakeholders to accept reforms that would, in due course, trim profits and slow the rate of increase in salaries and payments to well-heeled medical providers and manufacturers. As a practical political matter, reformers avoided spelling out clear, immediate costs to be borne by well-organized stake-holders, because this would convert them from supporters of reform to loud opponents. Instead, those who fashioned and enacted Affordable Care inserted into the legislation a multi-pronged framework for ratcheting down *future* payments, and delayed the start of many of these eat-your-spinach provisions. Reformers calculated that big insurance companies, pharma-ceutical manufacturers, and hospitals would be fixated on immediate opportunities to treat new patients and use gov-ernment subsidies and would not react too harshly to the long-term prospect of lower prices and profit margins in the future. Politically, it worked. The question, of course, is whether future policy makers will remain steadfast about imposing the pain. We think they will and explain why in the next chapter.

If the enemies of health reform were on a baseball team, they would be cut. Their shrill warnings since the passage of Affordable Care that the law would reduce insurance coverage, spike premiums, explode the budget, and sock Middle America with huge new taxes have all been proven demonstrably wrong. This is not an opinion; it comes from a number of non-partisan, data-rich studies by impeccable sources.

When all is said, the promise of health reform—as spelled out in the text of the 2010 Affordable Care legislation and affirmed by the Supreme Court—amounts to a very good deal for the great majority of Americans and for the country as a whole. The benefits provide security and lower premiums for already-insured Americans, plus new coverage for the uninsured and those who have skimped on much-needed medical care because they cannot afford it (even with some insurance). All of this does cost real money, but Congress wrote a law that asks for the tab to be largely covered by the most affluent and by the booming health care industry. The reforms are "paid for" in terms of the future national budget, and if they all work out as intended, they will give a boost to jobs, growth, and efficiency in the economy.

Sounds good. All that remains is to ensure that the reform law survives as all of its provisions are carried fully into effect.

5

WILL HEALTH REFORM SUCCEED?

"It ain't over 'til it's over." The wisdom of Yogi Berra obviously applies in his own world of sports, where shocking reversals—sudden or protracted—can undo seemingly inevitable victories, not to mention certain defeats. Driving toward the end zone in the final seconds of a tie game and well within field goal range, the 2009 Vikings appeared on the road to the Super Bowl, when Brett Favre hurled an interception and the Saints went on to win in overtime. Up by three games to zero, and ahead 4 to 3 in the ninth inning of game four in the 2004 American League Championship series, the New York Yankees let the Boston Red Sox come from behind to win that game—and then lost again to the Sox in game five…game six…and game seven. And of course in Super Bowl XLIX the Seattle Seahawks saw their hopes dashed by a last-minute interception in the end zone by an obscure rookie New England cornerback. Similar reversals happen in politics, as became evident first to Democrats, and then to Republicans, in the days and months following Scott Brown's surprise upset in the January 2010 Massachusetts Senate race.

Comprehensive health reform triumphed in the United States on March 23, 2010, didn't it? Wasn't the battle about reform finally settled when President Obama signed the Patient Protection and Affordable Care Act into law (followed by the Health Care and Education Reconciliation Act a week later)? Actually, no. Even with landmark legislation signed, sealed, and delivered, fights about reform have gone on and on—and will keep raging for years to come. Almost every outcome remains possible: substantial reversal, protracted defeat, or long-term success.

Reversal is much more difficult in the wake of two Supreme Court decisions that affirm the legal framework of the Affordable Care legislation—the June 28, 2012, decision that the law is constitutional and the June 25, 2015 ruling upholding subsidies that allow lower-middle-income Americans to buy affordable private health insurance on state exchanges established by the federal government. By 2017, twenty to thirty million Americans will have gained insurance coverage, even as all Americans continue to enjoy new insurance protections. Perhaps the health reform law could still be stalled or fundamentally revised if future elections bring a Republican sweep of the White House and both chambers of Congress, but politicians aiming to make fundamental changes would need to take away or weaken the benefits many Americans have gained. Short of repeal or fundamental revisions, the game will be protracted, and only after years of maneuvering and political arguments will it become clear whether the core promises of Affordable Care have been fully realized and the law has succeeded in extending insurance coverage to nearly all Americans, while also limiting price increases for everyday people and making the national cost of health care manageable.

In accord with the law, promised new benefits have taken effect, especially since major extensions of new insurance coverage started in 2014. Each step of the way requires spelling out new rules for health care providers, patients, insurance companies, employers, and businesses involved in supplying goods and services to America's enormous health care sector. Both federal and state administrators have been negotiating these rules amid pushes and pulls from all the stakeholders. Political controversies never end. Every group with profits or benefits at stake deploys lobbyists to influence legislators and runs ads to persuade Americans of their clashing perspectives. In legislative halls and recurrent elections, Republicans and Democrats fight

over repealing, changing, or carrying through the planned provisions. Heated debates over health reform were a centerpiece
of the 2010 mid-term elections that swept Republicans into
office and appeared again in the 2012 and 2014 elections.
Debates are likely to continue through 2016 and beyond.

TIMELINE FOR IMPLEMENTATION OF AFFORDABLE CARE PROVISIONS

2010   *An End to Rescission*: Insurance companies will no longer
be able to rescind coverage when you get sick.

Better Coverage for Young People: Children can stay on their
parents' plans until age 26. Insurance companies will no
longer be able to deny coverage to children because of
their "preexisting conditions."

"Doughnut Hole" Rebate: Provide a $250 rebate to Medicare
beneficiaries who reach the Medicare Part D coverage
gap, the first step in a process that will gradually close
the gap in prescription-drug coverage that had required
many seniors with significant prescription costs to pay
high amounts out-of-pocket every year.

Small Business Tax Credits: For small businesses that offer
health insurance to their employees, tax credits will offset
up to 35% of the employer contribution.

Expansion of Medicaid: States are given the option of
extending Medicaid to all American citizens and legal
residents ineligible for Medicare and earning less than
133% of the federal poverty line. Expansion must be
complete by 2014; the federal government will offset
states' costs for new enrollees.

Temporary High Risk Pool: People with preexisting conditions unable to find insurance are eligible to join the high-
risk pool and receive subsidies to make premiums
affordable.

2011   *Better Coverage for the Elderly*: Americans on Medicare will
no longer pay deductibles and other costs for recom-
mended preventive services.

2012   *Consumer Protections*: New standards will govern how insurers provide information about different plans, allowing consumers to comparison shop more easily.

2014   *Expansion of Coverage*: Credits and subsidies to low- and middle-income families kick in to offset costs of health insurance. Businesses with 50 or more employees are required to offer health insurance or pay a penalty. All U.S. citizens must have qualifying health insurance, with exceptions for those with religious objections or financial hardship (despite public subsidies).

Health Care Exchanges: Will be up and running in all states and regions, to allow self-employed, uninsured individuals, and small businesses to shop for insurance in new marketplaces providing consumers with better information about competing health plans and different levels of coverage.

Ending Annual and Lifetime Limits: Insurers will no longer be able to cap coverage based on an annual or lifetime limit, protecting the insured from losing coverage when their medical expenses are highest.

Ending Preexisting Condition Exclusions: Insurers can no longer deny coverage to adults because of preexisting conditions.

Shorter Waiting Periods: Waiting periods for coverage can last no more than 90 days.

That it ain't over—by a long shot—is sure to be dismaying to some. But none of us should be surprised. Landmark laws don't just mark the end of political struggles—they also start new ones. And even the most beloved and successful social programs in U.S. democracy have taken time to work out. The 1935 blueprint for Social Security was profoundly incomplete (it excluded most working women and about 80% of African Americans in parts of the South). Social Security had its financial provisions substantially revised in 1939, experienced life-threatening interruptions in scheduled taxes and benefits during World War II, and did not really become taken-for-granted until the period between the early 1950s and the mid-1970s, when taxes resumed and new beneficiaries and enhanced benefits were added. The implementation of Medicare was initially dominated by profit-seeking physicians and hospitals, until mid-course adjustments gave federal regulators greater leverage over rising costs. Political time now moves more quickly, so Affordable Care may become entrenched within a decade. Still, the 2010 enactments called for years of tricky implementation through an unfolding series of regulations, subsidies, taxes, and tax breaks—with fifty states as well as federal agencies involved, not to mention the need for partial reaffirmations in annual federal budgets along the way.

How are citizens to keep track of the complex maneuvers and clashing arguments? No one can predict the future (that is Yogi's point, after all), but we can lay out what is at stake and consider some possible scenarios. We start with the already highly public lawsuits that were largely unsuccessful before the Supreme Court, and then turn to ongoing quieter, more protracted negotiations that are likely to matter more in coming months and years. Every American should know the stakes—why it makes a difference how officials bargain with insurance companies and doctors and why it matters which party wins elections. Health reform holds a lot of promise for Americans and the U.S. economy. Yet the promise can be realized only after a lot of hard work, and only if people committed to making the new system effective manage to hold their own in ongoing battles.

HEALTH REFORM SURVIVES BIG LEGAL CHALLENGES

Before the ink was dry at the White House signing ceremony, the National Federation of Independent Businesses joined with conservative officials from (ultimately) 26 states to file cases in the federal courts arguing against the constitutionality of Affordable Care as a whole and against key provisions of the law.

Like gladiators suiting up for the next big match, lawyers, foundations, and advocacy groups on the right and left had been preparing for some time to argue legal cases about health reform. Reform opponents were outfitted by conservative organizations including the Heritage Foundation. Anticipating post-enactment challenges, the authors of Affordable Care legislation crafted in 2009 and early 2010 what they hoped would be bulletproof provisions, using legal analyses provided by the Congressional Research Service and grantees of the Robert Wood Johnson Foundation. Affordable Care was anchored in what its authors considered the sturdiest constitutional grounds and incorporated provisions that explicitly invoked the constitutional authority of Congress as affirmed in previous Supreme Court rulings. Although reform opponents energetically pressed their cases, they fought on the constitutional grounds chosen by health care reformers. The ultimate majority decision by the Supreme Court in June 2012 generally followed what we and other analysts of the legal and policy issues had predicted.

Soon after President Obama signed Affordable Care into law in March 2010, opponents argued legal challenges along three lines, none of which was finally accepted by majorities in three of the four federal appellate courts or in the Supreme Court's 2012 ruling. For starters, opponents urging outright nullification claimed that Affordable Care violates the Tenth Amendment to the U.S. Constitution, which states that powers "not delegated to the United States by the Constitution, nor prohibited by it to the States, are reserved to the States." Idaho was the first of a number of states to pass a law that sought to nullify the new federal law by declaring its residents "free to choose or decline to choose any mode of securing health care services without penalty or threat of penalty."[1] Although it was red meat for angry conservatives, this legal strategy utterly failed because the supremacy of federal law is longstanding. The Founders adopted Article IV in 1787 to establish the U.S. Constitution and federal laws as the "supreme Law of the

Land"; the Civil War and later battles over racial segregation defeated claims that states' rights are preeminent; and, more recently, federal courts have struck down state laws seeking to void Medicaid rules requiring payment for abortion in cases of rape and incest. Over the past half century, federal courts all the way up to the Supreme Court have routinely rejected Tenth Amendment challenges to federal laws.

A second line of legal attack initially also appeared to rest on tenuous grounds but in the end led to an important modification of federal authority to implement the Medicaid provisions of the Affordable Care Act. Bill McCollum, Florida's Republican Attorney General and a 2010 gubernatorial candidate, filed a lawsuit supported by nearly two dozen other states that challenged Affordable Care's call for the establishment of state-level health insurance exchanges and requirements for the expansion of Medicaid, calling these "an unprecedented encroachment on the sovereignty of the states." The major federal courts generally rejected these arguments; the Supreme Court affirmed the constitutionality of the insurance exchanges and the provision of new federal funds for the expansion of Medicaid to adults with incomes up to 138% of the federal poverty level beginning in 2014. But the Court did pull some teeth from the Medicaid provision—under the majority ruling, the federal government is barred from withholding *existing* Medicaid funding from states that refuse to implement the Medicaid expansion slated for 2014 and beyond. The Supreme Court ruling left in place incentives to induce states to choose to sign up—generous new federal funding that hospitals and patients want in every state.

The third and most ballyhooed line of legal challenge to Affordable Care zeroed in on the constitutionality of the "individual mandate" rule, according to which Americans would, with some exceptions, be required to carry health insurance after full implementation of Affordable Care made it available at a reasonable price to most people. This line of attack, constantly debated in the media, turned out to be much ado about almost nothing. Reform opponents charged Congress lacked the authority to require individuals to obtain health insurance or pay a fine if they declined.

But the reformers who wrote the Affordable Care legislation were ready to defend the mandate provision in various ways. First, they preempted legal assaults in 2009 and 2010 by designing the individual mandate to allow exceptions for people who cannot afford insurance or who have religious objections. The next line of defense consisted of two legal arguments by the Obama administration to persuade the Supreme Court about the constitutionality of the "individual mandate" provision—one of which struck home. Although the Supreme Court majority did not accept the argument that the mandate was constitutional under the authority of the federal government to regulate interstate commerce, a majority led by the Chief Justice accepted the constitutionality of the mandate as an excise tax paid to the Internal Revenue Service and thus anchored in the federal government's taxing powers as explicitly stated in Article I, Section 8 of the U.S. Constitution. Once a majority of justices accepted the individual mandate as an exercise of the taxing power of Congress, the survival of the Affordable Care Act was assured, even though the commerce clause argument was not accepted. Drafters of the law had wisely offered different justifications, any one of which would suffice. The bottom line was that the individual mandate survived intact along with an extraordinary body of new regulations to ensure that private insurers cover all would-be customers, including people who have health-threatening "preexisting conditions."

Big legal challenges to Affordable Care made for riveting political drama from March 2010 to June 2012 as they snaked their way through the federal courts to a knife-edge five to four Supreme Court decision to let the landmark law live on. In a decision that surprised many politicians and pundits who expected a straight partisan outcome, conservative Chief Justice John Roberts joined four moderate to liberal justices in upholding the core parts of health reform. As Roberts explained, "We do not consider whether the Act embodies sound policies. That judgment is entrusted to the Nation's elected leaders. We ask only whether Congress has the power under the Constitution to enact the challenged provisions."

What the Court did, in essence, was toss the struggle over Affordable Care right back into the political and electoral arenas where even the legal fights had been anchored all along. But the 2012 Supreme Court ruling did not eliminate attempts to get the courts to do what elected politicians could not achieve—eviscerate the Affordable Care Act.

Although the political fight over health reform remains front and center in elections, reform opponents also renewed legal challenges and, surprisingly, made it back to the Supreme Court in the 2015 case *King v Burwell*. With the law's constitutionality settled in June 2012, opponents took aim at its funding by challenging the distribution of tax subsidies to the millions of Americans who used state exchanges set up by the federal government. Their legal toe hold lay in one sub-section in a 906 page statute, which said that subsidies would be for purchase on exchanges "established by the state." Challengers argued that those words meant that federal subsidies could not go to customers in dozens of states where exchanges had been set up by federal authorities after state officials proved unwilling or unable to set up exchanges themselves.

But what might seem like a literal and obvious reading of part of the text of the 2010 law crumbled under the weight of well-established legal rules and precedents. Courts have said in the past that laws are to be interpreted in accordance with their overall aims, not just by focusing on a few words taken out of context. In an unusually strong June 2015 decision, six Supreme Court Justices affirmed that the Affordable Care Act always meant for subsidies to be available in all fifty states, and in doing so raised the bar for future conservative challenges. The Court declined to say that the executive branch has made universal subsidies available simply by offering its own interpretation of an ambiguous provision; instead the Court majority ruled that Congress always intended the subsidies to go to states relying on federal exchanges as well as to states that built their own exchanges. This means the issue is settled: even if a Republican President takes office in the future, he or she will not be able to deny subsidies merely by issuing a new administrative ruling. Congress would have to vote to overturn the subsidies—and take responsibility before the American people.

In short, despite some huffing and puffing about the sloppiness of Congress in writing and proofreading the text of the Affordable Care Act, the Supreme Court's 2015 ruling dismissed the challengers' focus on just four words. Following long precedents, the Court majority looked at the law as a whole and noted that universally available subsidies were necessary to make health insurance affordable in working insurance markets. Without subsidies, the Court noted, insurance markets in many states would go into a "death spiral," and that cannot be what Congress intended.

Of course, legal challenges to the Affordable Care Act have an effect even when they ultimately lose in court. Legal challenges by right-wing opponents of health reform have been part of an overall political strategy to mobilize partisans and convince worried voters that health reform is uncertain or dangerous. They have attracted media coverage and may have spread false public beliefs and stoked continuing grass-roots resistance.

In the lead in to the 2012 Supreme Court case, for instance, shrill warnings about a "massive new middle-class tax" supposedly imposed by the individual mandate amounted to fabrications not unlike the false scary claims about "death panels" deployed in the 2010 elections. In truth, the mandate applies only to a small number of Americans out of each 100, only to people who do not have health insurance through work or a government program, or who cannot afford to purchase coverage with help from generous tax credits. There are exemptions from the mandate for people who have religious objections or who cannot afford a plan. And here's the real kicker: the Affordable Care Act does *not* classify the failure to obtain insurance as a crime, and the Internal Revenue Service is not allowed to impose liens or levies on people who do not comply. The fine itself is small, and compliance is basically voluntary. This is the truth of the matter, but it did not prevent challenges to the individual mandate from shaping false media coverage over the course of several years, perhaps in ways advantageous to Republicans.

As for the most recent Supreme Court ruling, Republican leaders publicly bemoaned the 2015 decision but the truth is that it saved the GOP from a no-win explosion its own extreme right-wingers tried to ignite by taking away as benefits that millions of Americans (including rank and file Republicans) were already enjoying. Had the Court cut off many subsidies, millions of Americans who can now afford to buy private health plans in states ranging from Texas and Florida to Ohio and Wisconsin would have suddenly faced the loss of coverage—and losses of that sort make voters angry much more than potential gains make them happy. Non-Tea Party Republican officeholders and leaders in Chambers of Commerce in many states where subsidies were at issue were surely relieved when the Supreme Court left them in place. The ruling may have disappointed all critics of ObamaCare by leaving the President's main domestic policy achievement in place, unhappily for Republicans now and in the future. But it also signaled a setback for right-wing ideological bomb-throwers and gave a boost to Republicans who would like to get on with the business of winning government power to serve practical business interests.

CAN GOVERNMENTS BESET BY LOBBYISTS MAKE REFORM WORK?

As the legal and political battles rage on, the implementation of Affordable Care is proceeding apace. Amid lawsuits pushed by loud advocates and debated endlessly on cable TV, the truly high-stakes struggles have been going on less visibly in fifty state capitals and in the halls of the Department of Health and Human Services charged with making Affordable Care work on the ground. Legislative provisions require specific interpretation, and rules must be issued in Washington, DC, and by state governments to guide the behavior of insurance companies, health care providers, and businesses and citizens.

Of course, national and state-level public officials have not operated in a vacuum. Teams of well-connected lobbyists are squaring off against officials in the Obama administration and in state capitals. The lobbyists represent stakeholders determined to win lenient rules, even to the point of quietly reversing decisions they apparently lost when Affordable Care bills first made their way through Congress. In many instances, Congress gave in to pressures to word key provisions vaguely rather than strictly. This often happens with controversial legislation, and, as everyone knows, it opens the door to later, behind-the-scenes efforts to interpret the law in ways particular stakeholders find advantageous.

Hundreds of behind-the-scenes battles over interpretations and application of Affordable Care provisions are highly consequential for patients, employers, and of course for all the businesses involved in health care. Public servants sometimes find solutions that strike a middle way or give advantages to everyone. But often there have been zero-sum trade-offs. For example, not everyone can win when at least 80% of insurance premiums must be spent on necessary care. Insurance executives want a loose interpretation to protect money for their high pay, but reformers want a strict definition to further a core promise of health reform—widening access to better medical care at lower cost. More generally, if the Obama administration or state officials excessively accommodate insurers and the medical manufacturing industries—allowing them to continue business as usual with more money thrown in—then Affordable Care's new framework for cost controls will not work. Fewer resources would flow into actual patient care or improvements in quality and access, and patients and businesses would continue to face escalating costs.

Each interpretive battle seems small, but the overall pattern will eventually take shape in one direction or another. If, after some years, costs for patients and employers are very high and quickly rising, or if the quality of care suffers, that could generate public disappointment and fuel backlashes against the health reform law and its backers. On the other hand, if the Obama administration stands up to the special interests, health reform may do better overall—but there will still be a lot of political outcries from stakeholders who are asked to accept slightly lower profits and devote more of their resources to actual health care. Everyone should realize that there are continuing political issues either way. Outcries from privileged stakeholders may be a sign of progress for effective public regulation, not a sign of failure.

Even as special interests deploy their considerable firepower to rig implementation, a hidden truth lurks behind all the maneuvering. The very fact that insurance companies, employers, health care providers, and medical-equipment makers are lobbying and negotiating means that they implicitly realize the law is here to stay. In truth, many stakeholders in health care did not want Affordable Care to be thrown out by the courts, and they do not support continuing moves toward outright repeal in Congress. Supporters of Affordable Care—like the lead representatives of doctors and hospitals—pressed the courts to uphold health reform; and even groups that had originally opposed the legislation, like the insurance lobby, did not advocate for declaring the Act unconstitutional in 2012. In 2015, insurance companies certainly did not want premium subsidies assisting millions of their customers to be removed by the Supreme Court.

A new reality on the ground is unfolding as doctors and hospitals care for new paying patients, medical manufacturers enjoy new sales and profits, and insurers reconfigure their business models to conform, more or less wholeheartedly, to new rules of the insurance game. Stakeholders are gradually realigning their interests and behavior within the refashioned health system, unleashing new political dynamics that are familiar to students of American politics. Quiet cooperation is emerging where new policies are distributing subsidies to targeted insiders—as happens, for example, through insurance exchanges governed, in part, by insurers and other stakeholders. Reform is also spurring public competition to reap benefits and avoid burdens, competition that pits, for example, large against small insurers and medical specialists against general practice groups.[2]

As stakeholders invest more and more in making it all work, they become a bulwark against repeal or fundamental revisions. That happens when powerful interests manage to get interpretations of rules they like—and it can even happen when they don't totally like the new rules but get used to them or fear worse outcomes should a political battle be reopened. For instance, Republican control of Congress is producing unease among private insurers about ultra-conservative efforts to rescind much of Affordable Care, especially if those efforts threaten to leave in place popular new regulations—such as the requirement that insurance companies accept individuals with preexisting conditions—while trimming or eliminating the subsidies and tax credits that assure millions of new customers for private health insurance plans. Although Republicans and some Democrats might support a roll-back of funding, Republicans are unlikely to achieve the 60-vote margin in the Senate needed to repeal all of Affordable Care. This would leave regulations on insurance companies in force, while fewer customers would be able to afford their plans if subsidies were trimmed. In that scenario, Republican Party politics would devolve into an internal civil war between ideological right-wingers and more pragmatically inclined business interests.

The truth is that a new U.S. politics of health care is taking shape. Profit-making businesses want predictability and a path to steady profits. Public officials charged with implementing Affordable Care are crafting new rules of the game that most stakeholders can live with, and, over time, the new arrangements are becoming reassuring and appealing to many Americans. Conservative all-out opponents of Affordable Care may kick and scream every step of the way, and in some states and policy arenas all-out opponents of health reform succeed in delaying or complicating implementation. But the Affordable Care Act is already a new reality delivering benefits to tens of millions of Americans. There is no longer much doubt that, in the long run, most of the key reforms will survive, producing better outcomes in health care than the nation previously experienced.

Who Decides—and What Are They Maneuvering About?

Teams of lobbyists are camped out in Washington because, as one insurance executive explained, there are enormous stakes in official determinations of the "new parameters and new marketplace rules." The law's prohibitions against denying coverage, placing financial caps on coverage, and tying coverage and premiums to preexisting conditions force insurers to "rethink how they are going to do business," and decisions about how to oversee prices and investments in actual patient care dictate profits in a range of health care industries.[3] Each time an administrative determination is made or revised, there is a lot to talk about.

For all of the scrappiness that Obama administration officials bring to these discussions, they are fighting with their hands tied in two important ways. First, and most basically, the Affordable Care Act by its legislative design relies on the cooperative participation of private insurers, medical providers, and businesses involved in producing goods and services for the medical system—and those economic heavyweights have ardent advocates in Congress and access to voters through the media. If the stakeholders necessary to carry through reform don't like what Health and Human Services officials decide, they make "end runs" to appeal to Congress or even to the general public. This fact of life in Washington, DC—that end runs going above the heads of agencies are always possible—prompted a former health policy advisor in the Clinton administration, a man with longtime experience in Washington, to counsel the Obama administration to "tone down its criticism of past opponents of reform," "garner stakeholders' support and investment," develop "cooperative relationships" with Congress and its oversight bodies, and deploy "professionally run communications shops . . . to communicate [with] . . . the press, opinion leaders, stakeholders, and the public."[4] Even when the Obama administration officials bargain hard, the rules they design generally accept the need for private insurers and other businesses to keep operating at a profit. Implementation battles erupt over degrees of freedom, consequential but far short of any Armageddon. Despite warnings from reform opponents about a "government takeover," the private sector continues to be central to U.S. health care as Republicans like Senator Grassley have privately acknowledged.[5]

A second way in which public administrators have their hands tied involves divided authority. True, the legislation for Affordable Care grants extensive discretion to the Secretary of Health and Human Services—provisions saying "the Secretary shall" are sprinkled throughout the law. But other federal government agencies are also given important roles, and the fifty states are assigned key responsibilities. Decision making, of necessity, cuts across agencies and bridges from DC to states with highly varied capacities, traditions, and political climates. Instead of clear lines of authority, the power to make pivotal decisions at each stage of implementation is often dispersed enough to create confusion or allow for determinations at cross-purposes. This longstanding pattern in the federally governed United States endures.

Within this complex policy-making environment, lobbyists are targeting their firepower on decisions by administration officials about several core issues. The law prohibits insurers from imposing an "unreasonable premium increase," without first providing justifications to federal and state government officials. Congress gave a green light to the federal executive branch to publicly call out excessive premium hikes but held back in giving it the power actually to block higher rates. As a result, insurers flagged by Washington have stubbornly stuck to their plans, leaving some consumers with inadequate protection from rate hikes.[6]

On another front, lobbyists for insurers have made some headway in persuading the Obama administration and members of Congress (including Democrats) to delay or weaken the planned reductions in payments to private insurers in Medicare Advantage.[7]

Still another source of conflict is over the law's requirement that insurers spend at least 80% of premiums on "clinical services" and "activities that improve health care quality" for patients (the requirement specifies 85% for the larger group market). When insurers fail to document this pattern of expenditures, they must send rebates to insured customers, which have already totalled nearly $2 billion. Crucially, even as the Affordable Care law accepts the need for profitability, it attempts to limit the portion of premiums and government subsidies that can be siphoned away from medical care and used, instead, to pad administration, beef up profits, or pay megabonuses to top insurance bosses. Of course, insurers do not like this, so they lobby administrators along with key Democrats and Republicans in Congress to exclude from the calculations payments to insurance agents and also to broaden what counts as "improving quality." For example, they want "improving quality" to include expenditures on technology, funding for call centers for nursing consultations, and support for bureaucratic "review" of medical treatments chosen by doctors and nurses. In short, insurers regulated by the health reform law hope to include a lot of their regular expenditures and established administrative apparatus in the definition of "quality" patient care.[8] In response, consumer advocates are insisting that quality be tightly defined by measurable benefits to individual patients.

A lot is at stake here. An insurance executive insisted that no other feature of the law would be more "influential in shaping the future of the health care marketplace in the United States."[9] One of the Obama administration's lead negotiators with insurers agrees and noted that this and other detailed rules "could have a greater impact on costs and coverage" than the public option promoted by liberals back in 2009 and 2010.[10] So far, the Obama team has held firm in important respects—for example, insisting on the billion-dollar give back—but has still given ground to accommodate lobbyists and their well-placed friends. Of course, future sets of federal administrators may cede even more ground.

Fifty States as Partners and Stakeholders

The Affordable Care Act rests on a distinctive model for federal-state action. It promises substantial discretion for states to design Medicaid for the poor and fashion insurance exchanges to allow patients and businesses to comparison shop for private insurance plans. States have considerable leeway to tailor health reform to their particular business conditions and political proclivities. In addition to broad grants of authority to experiment, states have received billions of dollars of federal funding to set up and operate new programs.

State choices are producing different outcomes, ranging from strong business regulations and encouragement for cooperative nonprofit insurance plans to generous accommodations for private insurers. Experimentation can give conservative states enough latitude to define and embrace reform as their own invention, as states such as Kentucky, Idaho, Utah, and Iowa have done. Republican and conservative Democratic governors are rejecting "ObamaCare" even as they embrace what they call their own states' versions of...ObamaCare.

Liberals often imagine that state leeway under federal programs will inevitably lead to less-effective and generous social programs. But the Affordable Care Act relies on a new form of progressive federalism. Federal officials have the ultimate authority to set floors and prod improvements in medical care for all citizens no matter where they live. And this matters, because, for instance, death among babies, a standard measure of community health, varies widely, from 4.9 out of 1,000 live births in Massachusetts in 2007 to 13.1 per thousand in our nation's capital and 18 per thousand among African Americans who happen to live in Oklahoma. The law encourages states to establish the new health insurance exchanges and meld insurance subsidies with Medicaid expansions, but in key realms the federal government is assigned the legal authority to step in when states have not acted or do not meet minimum standards. For instance, federal backstops built into the law guarantee that citizens in all states have access to insurance exchanges—even in the 34 states that refused to establish their own or needed varying degrees of help to operate one effectively.

Congressional progressives and members of the Black Caucus insisted on such federal backstops to avoid past patterns in which southern and some western states collected federal subsidies and then minimized benefits for lower-income families, many of them black or brown. Congressional liberals originally preferred a unified national insurance exchange, but Scott Brown's election to the Senate from Massachusetts made the argument moot when it froze in place the regulatory aspects of the 2009 Senate bill, including the provision calling for state-level officials to set up and run exchanges.

Reformers and concerned citizens are watching closely to see if states use federal subsidies properly to help patients and small businesses buy insurance on the exchanges. Special interests are deploying lobbyists across the country to maximize the discretion of states to conduct regulatory oversight wherever possible.[11] Capitalizing on conservative climates in some regions, lobbyists are pushing relatively weak state regulators and playing on divisions between governors and state legislatures. Everywhere, of course, stakeholders can appeal to politicians and administrators who, pragmatically, hope to protect their states' industries and the jobs they create. Employers and their allies repeatedly invoke the threat of job losses or business closures when they want politicians to change laws or rulings in their favor. Sensitivity to such economic appeals cuts across the partisan divide. In "liberal" Massachusetts, for example, state bureaucrats have a lot of capacity, yet they also want to support the profitability of the great hospitals and medical-device makers so prominent in the state economy. Similarly, Minnesota's congressional delegation, though led by Democratic Senators who support Affordable Care overall, blocks and tackles for the state's medical technology industry. The Minnesota advocates, like those from Massachusetts, push for lowering or even eliminating the levy on the medical device industry, even though that industry will see its business grow as a result of health reform.[12]

Special interests thus enjoy a lot of leverage when they look to shape decisions in many states—and they regularly try to have the states with the loosest regulations set the tone for all the rest. Consequently, in the regulatory area, a "race to the bottom" scenario remains possible in health reform, even though the federal government has quite a few "backstop" powers to prevent states from going AWOL altogether. What seemed like an obscure decision during the debate in Congress to assign extensive responsibilities to states may turn out to be one of the most consequential features of the Affordable Care story over the long run.

Nonetheless, the apparent advantages business stakeholders and their lobbyists enjoy at the state level come with a big disadvantage—business interests have to argue and push in fifty different political arenas. After all is said and done, economic stakeholders then have to adapt to many different regulatory regimes, abiding by complex, idiosyncratic rules that vary across the country. Over time, national or regional insurers and medical manufacturers may well become advocates for more uniform national standards, even as they exploit the safe harbors fashioned by lax state regulators in the short run. This is one of the key ways in which decentralization will reshape political battles: it may create new converts to national uniformity. But will the new converts press for rules that are relatively good for more Americans? Not unless they have to-and not unless the tone of effective health reform is set by states with the wisest and most effective regulators. Federal administrators will need to remain alert and active in supporting and spreading best practices.

On paper, the federal government wields the enormous power to herd the fifty state cats—power attached to money and regulatory authority, which is assigned in provisions of the Affordable Care law. The legislation creates new federal authority to oversee the insurance exchanges operated by states; it allows the feds to say whether private insurers are offering benefits that meet basic standards, and to set quality standards for other facets of the emerging health system. The federal government is also authorized to spend hundreds of billions of dollars to subsidize the expansion of insurance coverage and support a variety of special programs and pilot projects. Knowing that Washington has these powers and resources, state officials are paying attention—and looking for cues about how to do things in approved ways. But at the same time, the full deployment of formal DC powers is being hedged by the usual micromanagement and henpecking from members of Congress, who, in turn, respond to pressures from lobbyists representing businesses in their districts. Federal officials are themselves trying to anticipate which actions of theirs will provoke—or avoid—Congressional micromanagement.

How these dances within Washington and between Washington and the states work out will centrally shape health reform in the future—and potentially push things in various directions. In addition to setting up the exchanges, states have major decisions to make about Medicaid expansions to cover low-income people just above the poverty line. The 2010 law made it very difficult for any state to refuse to use new federal funding to expand Medicaid to the near-poor, because it was assumed that states would lose previous Medicaid funding if they refused the expansion. But in its June 2012 decision upholding the constitutionality of the core of the Affordable Care Act, the Supreme Court said that each state could decide whether to do the Medicaid expansion or not; states that refused faced the loss of preexisting Medicaid funding.

In a stroke, the Court made Medicaid expansion a political process, to be decided state by state—launching protracted struggles in most states. By the summer of 2015, thirty states had adopted the Medicaid expansion in order to make use of the very generous federal subsidies that relieve states of about 95 percent of the expenses for extending new coverage to the near-poor. But many conservatives are perturbed about having to contribute even a little bit of additional state funding to pay for health care for low-income people, and so powerful right-wing advocacy organizations have pressed Republican governors and legislatures in many states to refuse to take the new federal money to expand Medicaid.[13] Very conservative states entirely controlled by Republicans—especially Texas and other southern states—have gone along with the right-wing demand to refuse the Medicaid expansion. But quite a few states with Republicans in control of the governor's office or one or both houses of the state legislature have agreed to take the new federal funds to expand their Medicaid programs— and we expect that more and more states will sign on. States that refuse are watching federal dollars flow to other states; and their hospitals and other businesses are losing profits.

Bit by bit, governors and candidates for office make the "let's keep up with the Joneses" argument to get their own state to accept federal monies too. In recalcitrant states, the cost for hospitals, health-care providers, businesses, and taxpayers will continue to rise, because the federal health reform law mandates steadily declining payments to hospitals that used to receive compensation for the care they provided to uninsured low-income patients. The 2010 law assumed that Medicaid expansions would take up the slack in every state, so the 2012 Supreme Court ruling created a fiscal vice for hospitals in states that have not expanded Medicaid. In those states, more low-income people are still uninsured, and when they need care and appear for treatment, someone has to pay. Either hospitals must absorb the cost and, in some cases, face bankruptcy, or state governments foregoing federal funds have to make up the difference.

What Will the States Choose to Do?

We cannot emphasize enough that so many opportunities for states to make choices leaves open possibilities for varied outcomes in the structure of health insurance markets and health programs. For all the talk of "ObamaCare," the reality is that reliance on states to implement changes does *not* further any single model of health reform in the United States. Instead, we see states and health providers headed down a variety of paths, creating alternative scenarios. Some are shaped by conservative policymakers, while others are influenced by liberal or progressive forces (and, ironically, could make progressives happier in the end than they might have been if a very limited national-level "public option" had been written into the Affordable Care law in the first place).

Here are some of the paths states may choose to follow as they make decisions about exchanges and Medicaid.

- Although Congress expected most states to implement their own health exchanges to avoid "federal takeover," the reality is that only about a dozen states have fully constructed their own exchanges (with a few others working in active partnership with the federal government). California and Kentucky have proven quite effective in shaping their own insurance markets, but that is hardly typical.

- States with leaders unalterably opposed to cooperation in running exchanges leave their residents to sign up via the federal website called "healthcare.gov"—and many of these states have also refused to expand Medicaid. Some states may eventually take over aspects of managing their exchanges. But on the issue of Medicaid expansion, quite a number of states may be able to hold the line for some years, leaving about four to five million low-income people without affordable health coverage. Eventually, however, budgetary considerations and pressure from hospitals and advocates may force even the most reluctant very conservative states to reconsider whether they want to accept generous federal Medicaid funding.
- States are also planning to use new federal funds to carry through reforms in their Medicaid programs, as long as the results are deemed "comparable" to standards set in Affordable Care. They can do this by filing for a waiver from Health and Human Services that allows the state to opt out of certain federal rules. As long as they provide comparable coverage and prices, states may encourage Medicaid recipients as well to take part in a purely privately run health insurance system, as Indiana has done and Utah is discussing. Alternatively, states can encourage enrollments in nonprofit coops—or, in the future, they might channel enrollments into some sort of public plan.
- In administering the exchanges, Washington, DC, and many states are working out creative partnerships in which some states use the federal website while at the same time certifying and managing health plan participation, consumer outreach and other essential functions. Even liberal Democratic states like Oregon have opted to rely on a federal supported state-based exchange after their own efforts failed.
- The Affordable Care Act also authorized expenditure of up to $6 billion by July 2013 to seed nonprofit, member-run insurance cooperatives that would emulate the health cooperatives already operating in the states of Washington and

Minnesota. About two dozen co-ops (which cannot be sponsored by existing insurance companies or by state or local
governments) have been launched for the purpose of serving consumers and reinvesting profits to lower premiums
and improve quality. Coops have faltered in some states,
but flourished in others. Over time, this approach could
expand as consumers search for an alternative to the large
insurers that dominate the exchanges in most states.[14]

As the preceding overview of various state-level options
suggests, the implementation of Affordable Care leaves a lot of
room for states to experiment—and the day may even come
when many states institute public option insurance programs
that prove effective in reducing costs. Should progressive state-
level experiments prove popular and effective in delivering
good care at reasonable prices, they could set the stage for
future rounds of health reform across many states or at the
national level. We have already seen this kind of process at
work in North America: Massachusetts reforms set the stage
for the 2010 Affordable Care law, and decades ago in Canada,
pioneering provincial programs led the way to national reforms
establishing a single-payer system. In truth, affordable, effective health care is attractive to both citizens and businesses in
all regions. So any experiment that furthers this outcome may
end up serving as a model for imitation by others.

When we move from listing logical options and future possibilities to looking at progress so far, we see that state implementation of Affordable Care has (with some notable exceptions)
largely followed the usual partisan pattern these days. States with
Democratic Governors and legislatures—including California,
Oregon, Vermont, Maryland, and Connecticut—are on course
to put health reform fully in place. States with Republicans in
control of the governorship or running one or two legislative
chambers have often been cowed by Tea Party opposition into
dragging their feet. Yet many states with Republican governors have adopted Medicaid expansions and gotten involved

in running or regulating exchanges. Varied state administrative capacities and policy legacies, and the political and
business cultures of each state, are playing a role in shaping
decisions along with sheer partisanship. Not all Democratic
states look alike; and Republican states are taking increasingly
divergent paths.[15]

And some reforms quietly included in the Affordable Care
Act have taken hold almost everywhere. With little fuss, nearly
all states have accepted the Affordable Care Act's offer to
pay 90 percent of the costs associated with modernizing the
administration of longstanding Medicaid programs, stream-
lining enrollments and eligibility determinations. Decisions to
proceed with modernization have often been made by obscure
state administrators, yet they modestly add to Medicaid enrollments even in states such as Texas that have not accepted
further expansion to cover people just above the poverty line.

Overall, we are seeing the reprise of a very old song in U.S.
politics. Room for state-level variety allows different verses to
be sung by many voices. Some of the singing may turn out to
be badly off tune, from the point of view of anyone who hopes
for a harmoniously effective national health system, because
varied arrangements leave room for special interests to push
weak state agencies around. But at the same time, certain states
may produce beautiful harmonies—if they have stronger administrators, more cooperative stakeholders, and more imagina-
tive citizen advocates.

We cannot prognosticate in advance where the best outcomes
will occur, or know exactly what shape they will take. What is
certain is that the United States will not have a unified, adminis-
tratively centralized health system—at least not for many years
to come. Once the states make their choices, patients and businesses will have a chance to see how things work out in different
places. Already, states with exchanges that have not functioned
well are being pushed by officials and citizens to look for better
options. Perhaps, in the end, the highest quality approaches will
be widely copied—with states that achieve good quality care for

all citizens at a reasonable cost winning out, offering models and setting the bar for all others. That is the best possibility—and reform advocates are trying to spur state-level decisions that make such a "race to the top" more likely.

WILL COST CONTROLS WORK?

Realizing the potential of Affordable Care means eventually including all Americans in affordable, quality health care coverage. But it also requires that we get rising health care prices for consumers and the nation under better control in the future than they have been over the past several decades. Health care expenditures thus become a key barometer of the overall, long-term results of ongoing struggles between special interests and state and federal administrators. Five years after President Obama signed reform into law, health care spending has risen at only three to four percent per year—the lowest rate of increase in half a century—and premiums for private insurance plans have increased only moderately and less than originally projected by the non-partisan Congressional Budget Office. Of course, these achievements could prove transitory, because lobbyists are intent on weakening government controls on spending and premium hikes in order to bloat industry profits, just as they did decades ago after Medicare was enacted in 1965. Medicare's costs nearly doubled according to cautious estimates, until a newly rigorous payment system was launched under the auspices of Republican President Ronald Reagan.[16] Will the Obama administration, members of Congress, and state government learn the lessons of Medicare's early years and fend off the special interests by maintaining and strengthening effective cost controls?

High Stakes for State and National Budgets

The fiscal stakes in battles over cost controls are huge for federal and state budgets. Although the federal government is paying the lion's share of the bill for expanding health insurance coverage to lower- and middle-income Americans, state governments could be forced after 2016 to pay hundreds of millions more per year for expanded Medicaid—from $220 to $300 million more in Tennessee and $370 million more in Texas to over $500 million more per year in California.[17] Republican Senator Lamar Alexander warns that these new health care costs "will force governors to cut higher education funding and raise taxes and tuition," and California's top health-policy official insisted that the "federal government...account for the states' inability to sustain our current programs, much less expand."[18] With state budgets already under pressure, failure to fend off demands from special interests for relaxed cost controls could precipitate a fiscal crisis in the states and induce bipartisan backlash among fiscal watchdogs in Washington, DC.

High stakes are also evident for the national budget. Although the Congressional Budget Office estimates that the new health system overall will save about $150 billion in federal expenditures, the reality is that some of these savings are projected on paper, not yet delivered in real life. Realizing the savings requires vigorous implementation of Affordable Care's multipronged strategy to slow the rate of cost increases in health care. In particular, public officials working with stakeholders must make sure that insurers restrain price hikes and pharmaceutical companies deliver promised discounts. In addition, Congress must maintain planned limits on future growth in Medicare spending.

Budgetary improvements also require success in longer-term efforts authorized by the Affordable Care Act to reconfigure American medical care and encourage individuals to adopt healthier behaviors. New tax incentives and research on what works or doesn't work must be used to squeeze waste out of medical care. Authorities have to discourage doctors and health care facilities from marketing high-cost treatments that deliver few tangible benefits—and discourage all of us from demanding such wasteful treatments. This will not be easy in a society that highly prizes freedom, even to make foolish

choices. But "spare no cost" is unaffordable. Government officials are certainly not going to tell doctors and patients they
absolutely cannot have even the most wasteful treatments, but
something still has to be done to nudge health providers and
patients toward better choices. Change depends on a gradual
cultural shift toward honest information-sharing and incentives for health-care providers and patients to make wiser
choices about effective yet less costly treatments.

Here is the hard truth: Most of the steps to slow the rise of
health spending threaten to eat into the current profits made
by some sector or another of the vast U.S. medical industry.
Congressional delegations are already at work trying to protect
their state's interests by weakening regulations and reducing
taxes on insurers, care providers, and manufacturers of medical
devices and pharmaceutical drugs. Some of the backtracking is
partisan—as in Republican efforts to abolish the new, fiscally
tough Medicare payment board that is supposed to recom-
mend (not require) cost effective practices. But much of the
effort may be little more than old-fashioned bipartisan propiti-
ation of powerful interests in each state or congressional
district.

Without limits, independent research demonstrates that
medical providers, especially hospital systems that dominate
regions, are quite effective in extracting overly generous
payments from insurers, who pass them along to those paying
premiums.[19] The rejection of Medicare's model of rate regulation by the legislators who enacted Affordable Care surren-
dered—at least initially—the power to reduce the prices
charged by hospitals, physicians, and other providers. This
was a major omission, because not only the U.S. Medicare
system, but also national experiences in Western Europe,
Canada, and Japan show that rate regulation is effective in
reducing medical costs.

If medical costs in the wake of Affordable Care start to rise
appreciably, it won't be simply because government officials
are lax or incompetent. After all, federal and state officials have

budgetary skin in the game. A more likely culprit, if cost increases spike, will be successful efforts by the health care industry to persuade friendly members of Congress to subvert controls. Standing up to lobbyists to mete out fiscal tough love is a tall order for politicians. "It ain't over 'til it's over."

Some Reasons for Cautious Optimism

Although the battle to control rising costs will remain difficult, there are reasons not to presume the worst. For one thing, Congress has a reasonably good record of standing by its commitments to control Medicare budgets over the past several decades.[20] Much of the skepticism about Congressional follow-through results from misunderstanding the 1997 Balanced Budget Act and its poorly designed formula to automatically decrease Medicare payments to physicians. This formula ended up producing far sharper cuts than the Balanced Budget Act intended, which threatened to drive doctors away from treating seniors and prompted Congress to repeatedly approve temporary fixes during the Bush and Obama administrations. Interpreting these bipartisan "doctor fixes" as fiscal backtracking from the original intent is wrong, because overly sharp reductions were never the intent. Indeed, Congress stood by the lion's share of the trims in physician reimbursements planned in the Balanced Budget Act (four-fifths of the 1997 cuts have remained in place, reducing payments 17% below 2001 levels adjusted for inflation). Congressional steadfastness dramatically slowed increases in Medicare costs overall and contributed to the balanced federal budget achieved under the Clinton administration in 1998. Apart from the misunderstood 1997 case, the significant steps to slow Medicare's rate of growth enacted in 1990, 1993, and 2005 were implemented as intended.

Early signs hint at another reason for cautious optimism. Looming government budget deficits give both parties an incentive to support cost controls and avoid constant giveaways.

Current proposals for deficit reduction retain many of the tough cost controls in the Affordable Care Act, controls that may already have contributed to moderating the growth of Medicare's spending. Even ObamaCare opponent Paul Ryan, Republican chair of the House budget committee, accepts many of the spending cuts passed in 2010.

A third reason for hope comes from noting that a lot of scare rhetoric about health reform is misleading. Implacable foes may cry out that health costs are still rising, implying that Affordable Care is failing because it has not put a sudden, complete stop to rising prices.[21] But the framers of the law never promised any such thing. Legislators who voted for Affordable Care relied on nonpartisan budget projections that acknowledged health spending would rise in the short term as access is expanded to tens of millions of newly insured Americans. How could it be otherwise? Yet the Affordable Care law also passed the short run test for fiscal responsibility, because its inevitable increase in spending to expand coverage was *offset by new revenue and public spending cuts*. Over the coming decades, the law does not add to budget deficits or national debt and actually reduces the deficit, according to the best projections. The longer-term test is more challenging. Will the law help overall rates of increase in all U.S. health costs, public and private, to fall below what they were projected to be prior to the enactment of Affordable Care? That is where faithfulness to cost control provisions becomes critical.

A final reason for guarded optimism relies on an idea current in health reform circles for a long time: Once all Americans are included in health insurance and stakeholders can no longer make profits by dumping sick people or shifting costs, it will be easier for the states and the nation to think creatively about controlling costs while improving quality. The case of Massachusetts, which pioneered a system like Affordable Care, shows that a new political seriousness about prices and costs quickly follows from universal access. After absorbing criticism for lax cost controls during his 2010 re-election campaign,

Democratic Governor Deval Patrick became an advocate for a 2012 law that dictated cost-containment steps including the setting of a target for annual increases in health care spending.[22] That a Democratic governor would turn so forcefully toward supporting cost containment is no small step in a state with wealthy hospitals connected to influential private universities. Massachusetts has not solved the health cost problem, but the establishment of near-universal coverage in that state has pressured government officials to take cost control seriously and prodded powerful insurers and hospital executives to sponsor promising new strategies.

A similar dynamic will unfold over coming years at the national level. The salience of budget tradeoffs and the risk of deficits will pressure Democrats and Republicans alike to accept trims in payments to medical providers and manufacturers, even in the face of persistent counterarguments from lobbyists. It is worth remembering that Ronald Reagan—a strident opponent of Medicare's enactment in the 1960s—pioneered a substantial expansion of regulatory controls over provider payments in order to rein in rising deficits in 1983. Looking to the future, Robert Reischauer (former director of the Congressional Budget Office) proclaims himself "modestly optimistic" about slowing health care inflation, because "Congress and the administration will be looking for any mechanism or device that can hold down the growth of [health care] spending."[23]

Still, the bottom line is this: The effectiveness of planned cost controls will be determined not only or primarily by what is written into the Affordable Care law but rather by how faithfully and cleverly the prescribed structure is implemented amid shifting, gale-force political winds. As Americans learned to their horror in the Wall Street meltdown and the British Petroleum oil rig disaster, doggedly effective public regulation does matter. For such regulation to happen, we must put in place expert, loyal, and courageous public administrators— and not undercut them every time they try to do something in the public interest. Well-paid lobbyists are pressuring the

Obama administration, Congress, and state governments to pull their punches in establishing aggressive cost containment that, of necessity, limit payments to health care providers and contain profits collected by insurance companies and medical businesses. Will American citizens let the lobbyists push legislators and public administrators around, or will they encourage the President, the Secretary of Health and Human Services, and well-intentioned state officials to hold the line? The answer will determine whether the implementation of the new law can deliver the cost controls all Americans need.

WHY FUTURE ELECTIONS MATTER

Elections since the enactment of Affordable Care have pitted Democrats who are mostly committed to seeing health reform go forward against Republicans who are campaigning to repeal Affordable Care (and replace it with, at most, token adjustments to the health care system that prevailed in 2009 and earlier).[24] Enemies of Affordable Care took control of the House of Representatives in 2011 and the U.S. Senate in 2015 and are using their majorities to vote repeatedly to repeal or gut the law. A Democratic President and (from 2011 to 2014) a Democratic-run Senate have stood in their way. But future elections in 2016 and beyond will have much to say about how far the efforts of opponents can go.

Originally, the fiercest critics hoped the Affordable Care would end up with a fate similar to that of the short-lived Medicare Catastrophic Coverage Act of 1988.[25] That Reagan-era legislation imposed immediate fees on wealthy retirees to pay for eventual additional protections for all Medicare recipients. Opponents quickly mobilized against the new charges and turned a group of vocal elders—those whom the bill was designed to protect—against the law. It was repealed a year later, before it could go into effect at all. But the Democrats who enacted Affordable Care in 2010 learned lessons from the Catastrophic episode. Drafters of the act front-loaded widely popular features that started to go into effect in the first two years—millions of senior citizens received $250 checks (the first installment in the process of closing the "doughnut hole" gap in Medicare prescription drug coverage) and more than three million young adults signed up to stay on parents' insurance coverage until age 26. President Obama was reelected in 2012, and the Affordable Care Act managed to survive until its core benefits went into full effect starting in 2013.

As reforms roll out more fully into the everyday lives of Americans, some Republicans have modulated calls for repeal and started to give lip service to retaining or "replacing" some of the most popular parts of a law they claim they still want to repeal.[26] However, sketchy Republican "replacement" proposals do not preserve coverage for most of the tens of millions of Americans who now receive benefits from Affordable Care. And Republicans have not been able to explain persuasively how they would keep the parts of reform that Americans overwhelming support—such as the rules that insurance companies must accept customers with prior health problems—without also keeping the parts of the 2010 law that conservatives despise—above all, new taxes on the wealthy and the mandate requirement that most individuals sign up for insurance.

Of course the partisan clamor is not over. Many congressional Republicans and presidential contenders continue to make loud promises about repeal (or "repeal and replace," with replacements never specified), because the "Obamacare" label is unpopular with hard-core conservatives and Republicans who turn out to vote, volunteer in campaigns and write checks for candidates. Attacks on health reform also come from lobbying interests who want changes in taxes and regulations and are willing to contribute to candidates who help them.

Republican politicians appeal not only to their base and special interests in Washington but also try to scare senior citizens and attract their votes by making hyperbolic claims that Affordable Care "cuts" and threatens Medicare. This is basically untrue. Affordable Care trims subsidies for private insurance companies in the Medicare Advantage program but does not cut, indeed actually expands, benefits for Medicare recipients. But facts are not really the point when politicians try to scare elderly voters, as Tea Party Republicans have done with false claims about "death panels" in health reform.[27]

The 2010 and 2014 elections swept into office (or retained) large numbers of Republicans, giving the GOP control of Congress and states around the country. Denunciations of health reform furthered such outcomes, as did economic troubles and the predictable tendency for the "out-party" not holding the White House to enjoy boost in turnouts. Republicans effectively portrayed Affordable Care as a "budget buster" inimical to robust economic growth. And in the midterm contests, younger, poorer voters—the ones health reform will eventually help the most—did not vote at the same high rates they did in 2008 and 2012. Many of them have been discouraged by the overall economic situation and are not yet aware of their highs stake in health care reform.

Democrats tried to blunt the Republican assaults in the 2010 and 2014 election by reminding voters that Republicans want to "go back to the failed policies." This kind of effort may yield more fruit in 2016, a presidential election year, because more voters will appear at the polls, making the electorate younger and more racially diverse than it was in 2014. Millions of these voters will be benefitting from expansions of health insurance coverage. Furthermore, elderly voters may not be as frightened, because some of the benefits offered by Affordable Care have become concrete and Medicare plans have not been hurt. In fact, they offer new benefits.

In 2016, therefore, Democrats may retain the White House or seize the majority in one of the legislative chambers of the U.S. Congress. If either or both happen, the Affordable Care Act will flourish, free from Republican efforts to repeal or eviscerate it.

On the other hand, should Republicans win big in November 2016 by taking the White House and majorities in both chambers of Congress, they could be in a position to roll back or quietly undermine the implementation of Affordable Care—forcing changes in the legislative framework for reform. Certainly Republicans in this scenario would be able to cut funding for Medicaid expansions and reduce tax subsidies that make private insurance affordable for businesses and families. These are all budgetary steps that can be taken, with some difficulty, by majority votes in the House and Senate. But without sixty votes in the Senate to overcome a minority Democratic filibuster, it would be much harder for Republicans to repeal Affordable Care outright or remove the non-fiscal parts of it, such as the regulations governing insurance company practices.

What is more, should Republicans suddenly find themselves in full control of Washington, DC, they would soon confront political dilemmas and downsides in any effort to stop Affordable Care in its tracks. They might try, but not all regulations can be removed quickly and some cannot be removed at all. So Republicans would face a scenario in which insurance companies are still regulated—told to take all applicants regardless of "preexisting conditions"—even though new paying customers are not on the horizon, because Affordable Care subsidies are being reduced in GOP budgets. Stalling or defunding Affordable Care might quickly prove quite unpopular. By 2017, tens of millions of Americans would lose benefits and protections they already count on and would intensely resent their cancellation.

Political scientists have long known that majorities of Americans (including Republicans and the affluent) are operational liberals; that is, they like specific government benefits. At the same time, most Americans (including Democrats and the less affluent) are also ideologically conservative, when arguments about government versus the free market are posed in general rhetorical terms.[28] Although Republicans have lambasted "ObamaCare" on the general rhetorical level as expensive "big government," their efforts to repeal a law with many popular specific parts have not gotten very far and success will be even more difficult as time passes. Even happy talk about removing the individual mandate collides with the sober reality that this rule is a necessary complement to rules requiring insurance companies to cover people with health problems. That is why the conservative Heritage Foundation and prominent Republicans from Richard Nixon and Robert Dole to Mitt Romney originally embraced this rule. And this contradiction is not the only difficulty would-be Republican repealers will face if they gain the political power to move from rhetoric to action.

Tellingly, the American public has moved in the direction of supporting "keep it and fix it." The proportion that still insists on repeal has dwindled toward only a third of all Americans, though at least half of Republican voters are still pushing for repeal. What is more, when we move from overall assessments to specifics, majorities of Democrats, Independents, and Republicans are supportive of such key parts of Affordable Care as "stopping insurance companies from denying coverage," "letting children stay insured until age 26," and "expanding prescription coverage for seniors." Outside of Washington D.C., everyday people are ready for the political games to stop and for reform opponents to move on to other challenges.[29]

The Supreme Court's 2015 ruling discouraging future efforts to gut Affordable Care, plus the growing number of Republican voters and states taking part in the benefits of health reform, signal a new era. More and more GOP leaders will move toward the same sort of grudging adaptations they had to make to Social Security and Medicare/Medicaid, with pro-business interests pushing back against ideological purists. In Affordable Care Act politics, this shift has been underway in many states for some time, as Republican governors in Ohio, Nevada, Michigan, Indiana and beyond have parried ideological right wingers to find ways to accept the Medicaid expansion that so greatly benefits their white and black poor citizens and the bottom lines of their hospitals. Even in Washington, DC, we will see more and more Republicans throw in the towel on outright repeal.

WILL HEALTH REFORM WORK IN THE END?

Even though the Affordable Act is progressing steadily and outright repeal is a fading possibility, matters are far from settled for delivering significant new benefits for the vast majority of Americans to be paid for by taxes on the wealthy and fees from businesses. The U.S. political system gives disproportionate leverage to the privileged and well-organized economic interests—the very groups that Affordable Care designates to pay for improved health care for all of their fellow citizens.[30] The fat cats don't like it, and they are deploying their potent weapons to fight back—money for media campaigns, legions of lobbyists, and now, with the Citizens United decision by the Supreme Court, an unlimited ability to contribute to electoral campaigns. With every resource at their disposal, such groups continue to weigh in as regulations are written and enforced at the federal level—and also as rules for running and overseeing insurance exchanges are decided in the states. Even after the Supreme Court's historic affirmations of the basic constitutionality and core provisions of the Affordable Care Act, the enemies of comprehensive reform continue to mount smaller legal challenges. And they continue to go all out to elect Representatives and Senators and governors and state legislators who, if they cannot repeal the law outright, will nevertheless be receptive to making changes in taxes, subsidies, and rules that delay or undermine efforts to widen access and rein in spending for special interests. Even when spectacular repeal efforts fall short, much pushback happens out of public view, as it can appear technical and not easy to dramatize on cable news—even when the stakes are huge.

We will not know for a decade or more how far the pushback gets. The sway of the powerful may well produce a steady rollback of many of the specific ways in which Affordable Care helps middle-income and lower-income Americans. It is just too easy and tempting for public officials of either party to enact tax breaks for the rich, or adjust regulations and subsidies as demanded by well-heeled business interests. Each

little change will seem small enough for an individual legis-
lator, including a Democrat, to rationalize. But the little concessions to the status quo and to the rich and the powerful have
the potential to add up.

There are also rosier scenarios—either much rosier or somewhat rosier. Perhaps the landmark health reform law will not
only withstand attempted body blows but also dodge many of
the efforts to trim back taxes, relax rules, and reduce help for
everyday Americans. Vigilant citizens can help to hold the line,
yet key stakeholders are also more likely than when reform was
passed to prevent certain kinds of rollbacks. Affordable Care
rules say that insurance companies can no longer deny applicants because of "preexisting" adverse health conditions, or
charge them huge, surprise payments when they become sick,
or dump them altogether when they become costly. These new
insurance rules are so popular that no political party in power
is likely to be able to get away with going back to the pre-2010
status quo ante. Consequently, insurers who do not want the
rules without additional paying customers are ready to protect
public subsidies that enable millions to buy insurance. Another
powerful force for holding the line against rollbacks is AARP,
which seeks to protect improved subsidies for prescription
drugs and preserve help for nearly retired people who get laid
off and need to purchase health insurance on their own.

Finally, federalism also protects health reform, because conservative and liberal activists alike have won victories in states
or regions that they want to preserve. Conservatives have fashioned a "private option" for expanded Medicaid programs, for
example, while progressive reformers have furthered coops
and might succeed in setting up public options in certain states
or regions. Chamber of commerce and other business associations are also getting in the act to urge Medicaid expansions
and the establishment of exchanges, responding to pressure
from hospitals, doctors, and other components of the large
medical industry that, in the final analysis, need reform to
proceed.

The historic Supreme Court rulings in 2012 and 2015 ensure the law's survival in the long run, even if court challenges and partisan battles over particular regulations and expenditures continue for some time. The arc of history now bends toward health care for all—and greater efficiency in the system as a whole. In the months and years ahead, Democrats and supporters of comprehensive health reform have many battles to fight—especially to protect aspects of reform that help ordinary Americans, not just businesses. But the difficulties likely to face all-out opponents of Affordable Care are likely to be greater, even if they prevail in an election or two and manage to derail or deform implementation for a time.

Ordinary citizens will be conscripted into tough battles whether they like it or not, for some time to come. But in the end, Americans always turn out to value and support major social programs that help individuals and families gain basic security with dignity. Social Security and Medicare were enacted only after ferocious opposition on par with resistance to the Affordable Care Act, and both remained politically controversial for some time after initial enactment. But as they were carried through and the initial visions of reform were realized in practice, these laws became beloved and indispensable to most American families. Social Security and Medicare also encouraged older citizens, regardless of educational or income levels, to become more attentive about government; before these programs were established, seniors voted at about the same level as other Americans, but now they are the nation's most regular voters, vigilant about politicians who might mess with their benefits and rights.[31]

Health reform is now on course to join Social Security as an indispensable and widely embraced anchor of everyday life for large numbers of Americans. Pundits still focus on the challenges and controversies for ObamaCare, but from a broader historical perspective, its progress has been surprisingly fast and smooth. Reform is speeding forward, delivering benefits to millions that few career politicians can attack without paying a big price. In actuality, if not yet in the realm of partisan rhetoric, the Affordable Care Act is successful—and here to stay. Many conservatives fiercely opposed comprehensive health reform precisely because they feared its tangible programs would become popular and entrenched. They were right.

Despite the continuing right-wing clamor for repeal, health care in the United States will not go back to the way it was before March 23, 2010. Ongoing struggles over the full implementation of Affordable Care have quite a way to go, but we have already seen an irreversible shift in U.S. politics, along with historic expansions in the social rights of American citizens. Affordable Care is now part of the social fabric of our country and has opened a new era of social protection. When the United States considers further reforms, as it surely will eventually, lawmakers and a new president will have options that were not feasible in 2009.

In this concluding chapter, we have learned why Yogi Berra's warnings still hold, why it remains to be seen how fully the promises of the Affordable Care Act can be realized in a fiscally whip-sawed polity racked by divisions of class, ideology, and generational claims. A century-long quest for comprehensive health reform in the United States achieved an uneasy breakthrough in March 2010 and the implementation of reform has now helped tens of millions of Americans. But none of us who follow the politics of health care need worry that things will become peacefully dull any time soon. Americans who need affordable health care, and who want to keep trying to improve the provision of care and coverage at a reasonable price for the nation, have plenty to hope and fear, and much to do in the coming months and years. We will continue to live in interesting times, where each citizen's understanding, voice, and actions can make a difference.

GLOSSARY OF KEY PEOPLE, GROUPS, LEGISLATION, AND HEALTH CARE TERMS

1332 Waiver: New opportunity for states in 2017 to recast health reform toward a greater reliance on private markets or toward single payer or public option models. States may proceed if they convince the federal government that the changes they propose would maintain or expand core coverage without raising the cost to the federal government.

Affordable Care Act: *See* Patient Protection and Affordable Care Act.

America's Health Insurance Plans (AHIP): The leading lobbying organization representing health insurance companies, AHIP began 2009 by offering public support for reform before spending millions of dollars in 2009 and 2010 protecting industry interests by opposing reforms to increase competition or lower the cost of health insurance.

American Recovery and Reinvestment Act (ARRA): Better known as "the Stimulus" or the "Recovery Act," ARRA invested $787 billion in programs to jumpstart the economy and reinvest in American infrastructure. The law included emergency financial support, such as extensions to unemployment insurance, funding for Food Stamps and school lunches, and a one-time payment to Social Security recipients, as well as funding for health care and the expansion of health-related information technology. The law also invested in infrastructure, including roads, schools, hospitals, and the power grid. About one third of the cost consisted of over $200 billion in tax cuts for individuals and businesses.

Axelrod, David: With the official title of Senior Advisor, Axelrod is one of President Obama's most trusted strategists, both during his campaign and in the White House.

Baucus, Max: A Democrat from Montana, Senator Max Baucus leads the Senate Finance Committee and was one of the most influential players in health care reform.

Bending the curve: Term used by health economists to refer to reducing the rate of price or cost increases; a small decrease in the present can significantly reduce rising costs over time.

Blue Dog Democrats: A coalition of fiscally conservative Democrats in the House of Representatives who insisted that health reform not increase the federal budget deficit and favored compromise to reach bipartisan agreement with the Republican Party.

Boehner, John: As the Minority Leader, Boehner led Republican Party opposition to health care reform in the House of Representatives.

Brown, Scott: In a January 2010 special election in Massachusetts, Brown defeated Democratic candidate Martha Coakley for the seat of the late Senator Edward Kennedy. This political upset in a strongly Democratic state deprived Democrats of a filibuster-proof sixty-vote majority in the Senate, and encouraged Democrats to pursue a "reconciliation" strategy that avoided further Senate delays. *See* Reconciliation; Coakley, Martha; and Kennedy, Edward.

Cadillac tax: Excise tax on the most expensive health insurance plans. Senator Obama initially opposed a somewhat different and comprehensive version that Republican presidential candidate John McCain proposed during the 2008 presidential campaign.

Coakley, Martha: Attorney General for the state of Massachusetts, Democrat Martha Coakley was defeated by Republican Scott Brown in the race for the open Senate seat after the death of Senator Edward Kennedy. *See* Brown, Scott; and Kennedy, Edward.

Congressional Budget Office (CBO): A nonpartisan congressional staff agency, one of CBO's most important responsibilities is estimating the effect of legislation on the federal budget. The estimated cost of a piece of legislation is often called its "CBO score." CBO scores that show budget deficits can make it far more difficult to garner legislative support.

Cornhusker Kickback: Included in the Senate version of health care reform but removed before the bill became law, the Cornhusker Kickback gave Nebraska an extra $100 million in Medicaid funding to secure Senator Ben Nelson's (D-NE) support for the legislation that the Senate approved on Christmas Eve 2009. *See* Nelson, Ben.

Doughnut hole: A term for the gap in Medicare prescription drug coverage. Medicare beneficiaries had to pay the costs of medications between $2,700 and $6,154 (in 2009). Under the new health reform law, the doughnut hole will be closed.

Emanuel, Rahm: Former Senior Advisor to President Clinton and Congressman from Illinois's 5th District, Rahm Emanuel is now President Obama's Chief of Staff.

Filibuster: Forty-one out of 100 Senators can obstruct the passage of legislation by simply refusing to end debate and hold an up or down vote in a process known as a filibuster. Although the filibuster has been used in the past (it effectively delayed civil rights legislation for years before the 1960s), its use, or even threatened use, is much more common today. Filibusters regularly delay or prevent action in Congress, even when a substantial majority supports a measure, because a "super majority" of sixty is required to stop a filibuster.

FreedomWorks: A conservative nonprofit organization closely tied to the Tea Party movement and led by former House Majority Leader Dick Armey, FreedomWorks advocated strongly against health care reform.

Gang of Six: A group of three Democratic and three Republican Senators on the twenty-one-member Senate Finance Committee, the Gang of Six unsuccessfully sought bipartisan compromise on health care reform, consuming a number of months during the summer of 2009. The group included Democratic Senators Max Baucus (D-MT), Kent Conrad (D-ND), and Jeff Bingaman (D-NM) as well as Republican Senators Chuck Grassley (R-IA), Olympia Snowe (R-ME), and Michael Enzi (R-WY).

Health Care and Education Reconciliation Act: The reform of America's health care system resulted from two separate pieces of legislation that Congress passed and President Obama signed into law. The first—The Patient Protection and Affordable Care Act— became law when the House of Representatives voted on March 21, 2010, to pass the bill approved by the Senate on Christmas Eve 2009. The second piece of legislation known as the Health Care and Education Reconciliation Act was passed by the House and received a majority of votes by the Senate. Because it used the "reconciliation" process (as had Presidents Bush and Reagan) to make changes in the budget and taxes, it did not require sixty votes to clear a filibuster. This second law reconciled differences between the House and Senate legislation, and included several important changes to the legislation previously passed by the Senate, including larger tax credits and subsidies to make more health care affordable as well as new Medicare taxes on individuals earning more than $200,000 or families making in excess of $250,000. The bill also reformed the student loan process, increasing Pell Grants for low- and middle-income college students and paying down part of the budget deficit. Although the new health reform resulted from two distinct pieces of legislation, we refer to both pieces of legislation for simplicity as the Affordable Care Act (or ACA).

Health Care for America Now (HCAN): An umbrella organization representing more than one thousand progressive organizations, HCAN worked closely with the Obama Administration but also pushed for progressive health care provisions, particularly the public option. Member groups included unions like AFL-CIO and SEIU; civil rights organizations, including the NAACP and the National Council of La Raza; and left-wing advocates, such as MoveOn.org.

Health Insurance Exchanges: Under the new health care reform, consumers will be able to shop on health insurance exchanges for competing health plans that meet or exceed common standards. The exchanges will be administered by the states and will help arrange subsidies for small businesses and for low- and middle-income individuals, in order to make insurance plans affordable for them.

Ignagni, Karen: President and CEO of America's Health Insurance Plans, the lobbying group representing the insurance industry. *See* America's Health Insurance Plans.

Individual mandate: A part of the new health care reform, the individual mandate requires all uninsured individuals to purchase a health insurance policy or pay a small fine. Those earning below the poverty line or for whom insurance would cost more than 8% of their income are exempt from the individual mandate, as are those with religious objections or coverage through their employer, Medicare, Medicaid, or other government programs. Most Americans will be unaffected by this provision.

Kennedy, Edward: Serving for forty-seven years as a United States Senator from Massachusetts, Edward Kennedy was an ardent advocate of health care reform. He died in August of 2009 and was replaced in a January 2010 special election by Republican Scott Brown who ran on his opposition to national health care reform. (Both Kennedy and Brown supported the recent reform of the Massachusetts health system that served as a model for the national reform adopted by Democrats in 2010.) *See* Brown, Scott.

Lieberman, Joe: Joe Lieberman was the Democratic Party's Vice Presidential candidate in the 2000 election and has been U.S. Senator from Connecticut since 1988. He lost the 2006 Connecticut Democratic Primary following his support of the Iraq War before going on to win re-election as an Independent and caucus with Democrats in the Senate. During the health reform debate in the Senate, his support was necessary to achieve the sixty votes to stop the Republican filibusters. His opposition to two progressive provisions, the public option and the buy-in to Medicare for those 55 and older, led to their removal.

McConnell, Mitch: A Republican Senator from Kentucky, Mitch McConnell serves as the Senate Minority Leader, and spearheaded the opposition by Senate Republicans to health care reform.

Medicaid: Medicaid finances medical care for the very poor through federal funding that matches state expenditures. States administer the program and have some leeway in setting the rules; in the past, many excluded individuals with no children (even if very poor, with incomes below a quarter of the poverty line). The new health care reform extends Medicaid to cover all American citizens, including childless adults, with incomes up to 133% of the Federal Poverty Line (in 2009, about $29,000 for a family of four or about $14,000 for individuals).

Medicare: Medicare is the government health insurance program for those 65 or older as well as the disabled and those with end stage renal disease. Health reform expanded Medicare's prescription drug provisions to close a gap in coverage known as the "doughnut hole." In addition, reform removed subsidies to private insurers involved in the Medicare Advantage program and increased Medicare taxes on individuals earning more than $200,000 per year or families making more than $250,000 annually.

Medicare Catastrophic Coverage Act: Passed by Congress in 1988, this legislation aimed to help seniors pay for long-term care and some catastrophic health expenses not covered by Medicare. Its taxes on wealthy seniors provoked a backlash that unnerved Congress and led to its repeal in 1989.

Nelson, Ben: One of the most conservative Democrats in the Senate, Nebraska Senator Ben Nelson was the last Democrat to sign on to health care reform. To secure his vote in December 2009, Senate Majority Leader Reid added to the bill a special $100 million provision to cover Medicaid costs for Nelson's home state, known as the "Cornhusker Kickback." This special provision was removed from the final 2010 version of the legislation. Nelson also took steps to strengthen anti-abortion provisions in the 2009 Senate bill; and he tried, but failed in blocking reforms in student loans when such changes were bundled into the 2010 health reform legislation in the side car bill passed by majority vote. Nelson's influence was greatest when the Senate needed 60 votes to overcome the filibuster.

ObamaCare: Term most commonly used by conservative critics to refer to the Patient Protection and Affordable Care Act. In reality, President Obama only outlined general principles to guide Congress and did not offer a particular legislative proposal.

Office of Management and Budget (OMB): A part of the White House executive office, OMB helps the President manage the far-flung set of departments and agencies by producing his annual federal budget proposal, reviewing regulatory policies, and overseeing the development of legislation. OMB's analysis of fiscal costs was an important factor in the formulation of health reform. *See* Orszag, Peter.

Organizing for America: The organization succeeded the Obama campaign organization "Obama for America," and is run under the auspices of the Democratic National Committee to encourage grassroots support of the President's agenda.

Orszag, Peter: Peter Orszag was President Obama's first Director of the Office of Management and Budget and served until the summer of 2010. He was an influential figure in designing the Obama Administration's strategy for health care reform and advising Congress as it formulated health reform. Before joining the Obama Administration, Orszag led the Congressional Budget Office, and also served as an economic advisor in the Clinton Administration.

Patient Protection and Affordable Care Act (also known as the Affordable Care Act or ACA): The first of two pieces of legislation making up the 2010 health care reform, the Patient Protection and Affordable Care Act was passed by the Senate on Christmas Eve 2009 and by the House of Representatives on March 21, 2010, and then signed into law on March 23, 2010. The second piece of legislation— Health Care and Education Reconciliation Act—was passed by Congress and signed by Obama shortly afterward, reconciling outstanding differences between the House and Senate. Although the new health reform resulted from two distinct pieces of legislation, we refer to both pieces of legislation for simplicity as the Affordable Care Act (or ACA). *See* Health Care and Education Reconciliation Act.

Pelosi, Nancy: The Speaker of the House of Representatives, California Democrat Nancy Pelosi guided the passage of health care reform in the House. Her encouragement of a reconciliation strategy in 2010 was vital to the final passage of health care reform. *See* Reconciliation.

Pharmaceutical Research and Manufacturers of America (PhRMA): It is the lobbying organization that represents drug companies. PhRMA and Democratic leaders struck a deal in advance of health care reform that secured their support and agreement to accept reduced payments in exchange for protection against harsher measures. PhRMA's lobbying expenditure reached an all-time peak at more than $26 million in 2009.

Pre-existing condition: Prior to the passage of the new health care reform, health insurance companies could deny coverage to people who already suffered from an illness or medical condition (such as cancer). The new health care reform prohibits health insurance companies from denying coverage to individuals who had pre-existing medical conditions (this provision applies to children starting in 2010 and to adults in 2014).

Public option: The "public option" was a policy promoted by progressives and many Democrats to create a government-run health insurance plan that people and businesses could choose instead of a private plan. A national public option was not included in the final version of the 2010 health care reform legislation, though the new law makes it possible for states to choose to establish one or another variant of public options.

Reconciliation: In the Senate, where the need to assemble sixty votes to stop a filibuster frequently threatens to delay or prevent the passage of legislation, reconciliation is a process that allows budget bills to come to a vote and be decided based on a simple majority. Reconciliation played a crucial role in completing the 2010 health reform legislation. In 2009, health reform bills were passed by both the House and Senate, and Democrats expected to compromise the different versions in a regular conference committee held early in 2010, after which the finally adjusted health reform bill would go back to the House for majority vote and back to the Senate for vote by the same 60 members who supported the 2009 Senate bill. But after Scott Brown won the January 2010 Massachusetts special election for a Senate seat, Democrats no longer had sixty votes to overcome a filibuster. Instead, the House passed the 2009 Senate bill in March 2010, along with an additional reconciliation bill that adjusted taxes and benefits, in effect carrying through many of the compromises between the House and Senate that would have occurred in a regular conference committee. This reconciliation bill (called a "sidecar") was then sent to the Senate for enactment by majority vote, getting around the new obstacle created by Brown's arrival as the forty-first Republican. In the past, the same kind of majority-vote reconciliation strategy had been frequently used for bills with a significant budgetary impact, including the Bush Administration's tax cuts. *See* Filibuster and Sidecar.

Recovery Act: *See* American Recovery and Reinvestment Act (ARRA).

Reid, Harry: As Majority Leader of the Senate, Nevada Senator Harry Reid corralled a difficult coalition of conservative and progressive Democrats to achieve final passage of health care reform without the support of a single Republican and despite the constant threat of filibusters. *See* Filibuster.

Rescission: Before the passage of health care reform, health insurance companies canceled the policies of Americans who got severely sick—a process called rescission. Under health care reform, rescission is prohibited.

Romney, Mitt: As Governor of Massachusetts, Republican Mitt Romney successfully led the 2006 fight to pass health reform for his state, establishing a framework that became the model for the national health care reform passed by the Democrats in 2010.

Sebelius, Kathleen: Former Governor and former Insurance Commissioner of Kansas, Kathleen Sebelius is currently serving as the Secretary of Health and Human Services and is leading the effort to implement the Affordable Care Act.

Service Employees International Union (SEIU): A union with 2.2 million members, SEIU was a key advocate of health care reform.

Sidecar: Nickname given to the Health Care and Education Reconciliation Act passed along with the Affordable Care Act in March 2010. It was passed in the Senate using the "reconciliation process" that required a simple majority, circumventing the filibuster's requirement of sixty votes. *See* Filibuster and Reconciliation

Single payer: In order to provide universal health coverage, single payer systems use a unified public payer (e.g., the provincial governments in Canada) to pay the bills for people's health costs, rather than processing payments through a patchwork of private insurers. Single payer, unlike the public option, was not a prominent part of the U.S. health care reform debate during 2009 and 2010, even though the Affordable Care Act allows states to establish single payer systems if they choose. *See* Public option.

Snowe, Olympia: Moderate Republican Senator from Maine and a member of the "Gang of Six" and courted by President Obama and Congressional Democrats to give a "bipartisan" vote to health reform. She voted for the Senate Finance bill, but opposed all further reform legislation.

State Children's Health Insurance Program (SCHIP): The publicly funded insurance program for children in low-income families who earn too much to qualify for Medicaid.

Stupak Amendment: Written by Representatives Bart Stupak and Joseph Pitts, this amendment to the House version of health care reform prohibited the use of federal funds to pay for abortion coverage, either through a public option or subsidies in the health care exchanges. The Senate adopted a provision that more closely conformed to the Hyde Amendment that barred federal funding of abortions, which was included in the final health care reform bill.

Superdelegate: In the presidential nomination processes run by the Democratic and Republican parties, superdelegates are delegates to the national conventions who are selected not directly via election in primaries or caucuses, but through designation on account of their status as elected officials and senior party leaders.

Tea Party: A loose coalition of conservative activists, the Tea Party was a major media presence in 2009 and 2010, opposing the Obama Administration's agenda, including health care reform.

NOTES

Introduction

1. Sheryl Gay Stolberg and Robert Pear, "A Stroke of a Pen, Make That 20, and It's Official," *New York Times*, March 24, 2010, p. A19.
2. Ibid.
3. In 2007, 62% of personal bankruptcies in America were the result of medical expenses., according to David U. Himmelstein, Deborah Thorne, Elizabeth Warren, and Steffie Woolhandler. "Medical Bankruptcy in the United States, 2007: Results of a National Study," *American Journal of Medicine*, 122 (8) (2009): 741–746.
4. Kaiser Family Foundation, "Summary of New Health Reform Law," *Focus on Health Reform*, April 21, 2010.
5. Kaiser Family Foundation, "Health Insurance Coverage for the Total Population" 2013. http://kff.org/other/state-indicator/total-population/
6. Department of Health and Human Services, "Health Insurance Coverage and the Affordable Care Act," May 5, 2015. http://aspe.hhs.gov/health/reports/2015/uninsured_change/ib_uninsured_change.pdf (accessed July 21, 2015).
7. Department of Health and Human Services, "Health Insurance Marketplaces." March 10, 2015.http://aspe.hhs.gov/health/reports/2015/MarketPlaceEnrollment/Mar2015/ib_2015mar_enrollment.pdf (accessed July 21, 2015).
8. David Leonhardt, "In the Process, Pushing Back at Inequality," *New York Times*, March 24, 2010, pp. A1, A19.
9. During the enactment of the new health care legislation in 2010, the Congressional Budget Office (CBO) estimated that it would produce a net reduction in federal deficits of $143 billion by 2019. Four years later, the CBO found that the law's costs were even less than it originally estimated and the ACA's reductions in the federal deficits were greater. Letter to Speaker Nancy Pelosi from CBO Director Douglas W. Elmendorf, "Cost estimate for the amendment

in the nature of a substitute for H.R. 4872, incorporating a proposed manager's amendment made public on March 20, 2010," March 20, 2010; Congressional Budget Office. "Budget and Economic Outlook, 2014–2024." February 2014. Washington, DC. Pub. No. 4869. http://cbo.gov/sites/default/files/cbofiles/attachments/45010-Outlook2014_Feb.pdf (accessed January 8, 2015) and "Updated Estimates of the Effects of the Insurance Coverage Provisions of the Affordable Care Act." April 2014. Washington, DC. Pub. No. 4930. http://www.cbo.gov/sites/default/files/ cbofiles/attachments/45231-ACA_Estimates.pdf (accessed January 8, 2015).

10. Massachusetts Institute of Technology health economist Jonathan Gruber, who advised both the Romney and Obama Administrations as they instituted health care reform, has called Romney "the intellectual father of national health care reform." Sasha Issenberg, "Romney Defends Mass. Health Care Law," *The Boston Globe*, March 30, 2010.

Timeline of Health Reform Events

1. Faiz Shakir, "Obama, 3 years ago: 'I will judge my first term as president on' whether we delivered health care," *Think Progress*, March 23, 2010.
2. The transcript of Barack Obama's acceptance speech is available through the *New York Times* Web site: http://www.nytimes.com/2008/08/28/us/politics/28text-obama.html.
3. "American Recovery and Reinvestment Act (ARRA): Medicaid and Health Care Provisions," *Kaiser Commission on Medicaid Facts: Medicaid and the Uninsured, Kaiser Family Foundation*, March 2009.
4. "Transforming and Modernizing America's Health Care System," *President Obama's Fiscal 2010 Budget*, Office of Budget and Management.
5. Lori Montgomery and Perry Bacon Jr., "Key Senator Calls for Narrower Reform Measure," *Washington Post*, August 20, 2009.
6. Sheryl Gay Stolberg, "'Public Option' in Health Plan May Be Dropped," *New York Times*, August 16, 2009.
7. Carrie Budoff Brown and Patrick O'Connor, "The Fallout: Democrats Rethinking Health Care Bill," *Politico*, January 21, 2010.
8. Gail Russell Chaddock, "With Scott Brown's Election, Healthcare Ball in Pelosi's Court," *Christian Science Monitor*, January 21, 2010.
9. Carrie Budoff Brown and Patrick O'Connor, "The Fallout: Democrats Rethinking Health Care Bill," *Politico*, January 21, 2010.

Chapter 1

1. Theda Skocpol, *Boomerang: Health Reform and the Turn Against Government* (New York: Norton, 1997).
2. "President Obama Speaks at Healthcare Summit," CQ Transcript Wire, *The Washington Post*, March 5, 2009, 1:41 PM.
3. Karen Tumulty, "The Health Care Crisis Hits Home," *Time*, March 16, 2009, p. 26.

4. Ibid. All quotes, including quotes attributed to the Assurant Web site come from the *Time* article.

5. Ibid, p.28.

6. Ibid.

7. Total uninsured, 18 and 64 years old. "People Without Health Insurance Coverage by Selected Characteristics: 2007 and 2008." U.S. Census Bureau, Current Population Survey, *2008 and 2009 Annual Social and Economic Supplements.* Revised September 22, 2009.

8. Ibid.

9. For an excellent overview and analysis, see Katherine Swartz, *Reinsuring Health: Why More Middle-Class People Are Uninsured and What Government Can Do* (New York: Russell Sage Foundation, 2006).

10. The following trends come from Hye Jin Rho and John Schmitt, "Health–Insurance Coverage Rates for US Workers, 1979–2008," Center for Economic and Policy Research, Washington, DC, March 2010, Figure 3, p. 18.

11. Tom Daschle, with Scott S. Greenberger and Jeanne M. Lambrew, *Critical: What We Can Do About the Health-Care Crisis* (New York: St. Martin's, 2008), p. 3. The figures refer to the situation in 2007 and come from the Kaiser Family Foundation.

12. As quoted in "Reuters: Wellpoint Targets Breast Cancer Patients for Rescission," *The Medical News,* April 24, 2010.

13. Ibid, pp. 4–5.

14. Kaiser Family Foundation, "Trends in Health Costs and Spending" (March 2009).

15. Ibid.

16. Walter Pearson, Head of the Health Division, Organisation for Economic Cooperation and Development, "Disparities in health expenditure across OECD countries: Why does the United States spend so much more than other countries?" *Written Statement to the Senate Special Committee on Ageing,* September 30, 2009.

17. It is difficult to measure the extent to which doctors practice "defensive medicine," ordering extra tests or procedures to protect against charges of malpractice. Although proposals are frequently made in Congress to limit doctors' and hospitals' liability in the case of medical malpractice (a policy proposal known as "tort reform"), the Congressional Budget Office has found that tort reform would reduce health care costs by only about 0.5%. Letter to Senator Orrin Hatch from CBO Director Douglas W. Elmendorf, "CBO's analysis of the effects of proposals to limit costs related to medical malpractice ('tort reform')" (October 9, 2009).

18. The following examples come from Daschle, *Critical,* pp. 32–34.

19. Robert Uithoven, as quoted in Greg Sargent, "Lowden's Campaign Chief: Everyone Has Access to Health Care—at the Emergency Room," *The Plum Line,* online blog at the *Washington Post,* posted May 3, 2010.

20. U.S. Department of Health and Human Services, "New Data Say Uninsured Account for Nearly One-Fifth of Emergency Room Visits," News Release at HHS.gov, Wednesday, July 15, 2009.

21. Reed Abelson, "Bills Stalled, Hospitals Fear Rising Unpaid Care," *The New York Times*, February 8, 2010.

22. A study of the more formally registered parts of this dance of shifting costs among a disparate set of payers finds that about a quarter of the cost of "uncompensated care" (not covered by the patient or his or her insurance) is borne by various private sources, another quarter by state governments, and about half by the federal government. See Henry J. Kaiser Family Foundation, "The Cost of Not Covering the Uninsured," June 2003, Figure 4.

23. For early decades, see Ronald L. Numbers, *Almost Persuaded: American Physicians and Compulsory Health Insurance, 1912–1920* (Baltimore: Johns Hopkins University Press, 1978); Daniel S. Hirshfield, *The Lost Reform* (Cambridge, Mass.: Harvard University Press, 1970); and Monte M. Poen, *Harry S. Truman versus the Medical Lobby* (Columbia: University of Missouri Press, 1979).

24. Lawrence R. Jacobs. "The Politics of America's Supply State: Health Reform and Medical Technology." Health Affairs. 14:2 (Summer 1995): 143–157.

25. Jacob S. Hacker, *The Divided Welfare State: The Battle over Public and Private Social Benefits in the United States* (New York and Cambridge: Cambridge University Press, 2002), pp. 221–243.

26. Lawrence R. Jacobs, *The Health of Nations: Public Opinion and the Making of American and British Health Policy* (Ithaca, N.Y.: Cornell University Press, 1993).

27. Helpful overviews from which the following draws include Hacker, *Divided Welfare State,* part III; Swartz, *Reinsuring* Health; and "America's Achilles Heel: Job-Based Coverage and the Uninsured," The Century Foundation, New York City, 2004; Henry Aaron and William Schwartz, "Painful Prescription: Rationing Hospital Care" (Washington, D.C.: Brookings Institution, 1984).

28. Medicare's reimbursement of medical providers was initially ceded to private insurers and especially Blue Cross and Blue Shield to create a "buffer" between the medical profession and government to prevent government intrusion. Although civil servants in the Kennedy and Johnson administrations recommended "direct administrative control" over government funds, Medicare in effect allowed providers to write their own checks based on loose definitions of "customary, usual, and reasonable" charges and, as predicted, costs skyrocketed.

29. Peter Orszag, Director of the Congressional Budget Office, "Growth in Health Care Costs," Statement before U.S. Senate Committee on the Budget, January 31, 2008. p. 3.

30. Quoted from the abstract to Mark Merlis, Douglas Gould, and Bisundev Mahato, "Rising Out-Of-Pocket Spending for Medical Care: A Growing Strain on Family Budgets," The Commonwealth

Fund, February 2006. See also Kathryn Anne Paez, Lan Zhao, and Wenke Hwang, "Rising Out-Of-Pocket Spending for Chronic Conditions: A Ten-Year Trend," *Health Affairs* 28(1): 15–25.

31. In 2007, 62% of personal bankruptcies in America were the result of medical expenses. David U. Himmelstein, Deborah Thorne, Elizabeth Warren, Steffie Woolhandler. 2009. "Medical Bankruptcy in the United States, 2007: Results of a National Study," *American Journal of Medicine*, 122 (8): 741–746.

32. Paez, Zhao, and Hwang, "Spending for Chronic Conditions."

33. Lawrence Jacobs, "1994 All Over Again? Public Opinion and Health Care," *New England Journal of Medicine*, Vol. 358, No. 18, May 1, 2008, pp. 1881–1883.

34. Our accounts of the election campaigns draw from John Heilemann and Mark Halperin, *Game Change: Obama and the Clintons, McCain and Palin, and the Race of a Lifetime* (New York: HarperCollins, 2010) and Richard Wolffe, *Renegade: The Making of a President* (New York: Crown, 2009).

35. Heilemann and Halperin, *Game Change*, p. 107.

36. Ibid.

37. Transcript of "New Leadership on Health Care: A Presidential Forum," Cox Pavilion, Las Vegas, Nevada. Saturday, March 24, 2007.

38. From a transcript excerpt reported by Mark Halperin, in *Time* magazine's blog "The Page," November 27, 2007.

39. Barack Obama, "Remarks in Bristol, Virginia," June 5, 2008, available at the Obama campaign Web site, barackobama.com.

40. Ibid.

41. Barack Obama, "Address Accepting the Presidential Nomination at the Democratic National Convention in Denver: "The American Promise," August 28, 2008. Available at the Obama campaign Web site, barackobama.com.

42. Video of the "Prescription" campaign ad is available at the official Barack Obama YouTube channel, Barackobamadotcom.

43. Jacobs, "1994 All Over Again?"

44. Chuck Todd and Sheldon Gawiser, *How Barack Obama Won* (New York: Vintage Books, 2009).

45. In April of 2009, 71% of Americans had a great deal or a fair amount of confidence in President Obama's handling of the economy. Frank Newport, "Americans Most Confident in Obama on Economy." Gallup, April 13, 2009.

46. "The Travails of Tom Daschle," *New York Times* editorial, February 2, 2009.

47. In his February 9, 2009, press conference, President Obama commented that the "Republicans were brought in early and were consulted. And you'll remember that when we initially introduced our framework, they were pleasantly surprised and complimentary about the tax cuts that were presented in that framework. Those tax cuts are still in there. I mean, I suppose what I could have done is started off with no tax cuts, knowing that I was going to want

some, and then let them take credit for all of them. And maybe that's the lesson I learned." White House press conference, February 9, 2009. Available at the White House Web site.

48. Lawrence R. Jacobs and Robert Y. Shapiro, *Politicians Don't Pander: Political Manipulation and the Loss of Democratic Responsiveness* (Chicago: University of Chicago Press, 2000). For analysis of elite manipulation through crafted talk and policy design, see Jacob Hacker and Paul Pierson, 2005. "Abandoning the Middle," *Perspectives on Politics*, Vol. 3, No. 1, pp. 33–53.

49. Todd and Gawiser, *How Barack Obama Won*, p. 44.

50. William Galston, "In Defense of Caution," *The New Republic*, November 4, 2008.

51. Peter Baker, "What Happened? The Limits of Rahmism." *New York Times Magazine*, March 14, 2010.

52. Quoted in Sheryl Gay Stolberg, "Democrats Raise Alarms Over Health Bill Costs," *New York Times*, November 9, 2010.

53. Interview by authors with Executive Branch Office on January 5, 2010.

54. Interview by authors with Congressional official on January 3, 2010.

55. Interview by authors with Congressional official on January 3, 2010.

56. Remarks by the President on the Fiscal Year 2010 Budget, February 26, 2009. Available at the White House Web site.

57. Jeff Zeleny, "Obama: 'Stars Are Aligned' This Year for Health Care," The *New York Times'* blog The Caucus, May 13, 2009.

58. Briefing by White House Press Secretary Robert Gibbs, July 13, 2009. Available at the White House Web site.

Chapter 2

1. Jonathan Alter, *The Promise: President Obama, Year One* (New York: Simon & Schuster, 2010).

2. Adam Nagourney, Jeff Zeleny, Kate Zernike, and Michael Cooper, "G.O.P Used Energy and Stealth to Win Seat," *New York Times*, January 20, 2010. Dana Milbank, "Obama vs. the liberals: Pass the tea to the left," *Washington Post*, p. A02, December 17, 2009.

3. Alter, *The Promise*, p. 399.

4. President Barack Obama, Speech to Congress, "Obama's Health Care Speech to Congress." September 9, 2009.

5. President Obama, "Obama's Health Care Speech to Congress."

6. Brian Stelter, "MSNBC Presses Obama on Campaign Promises," *New York Times*, November 15, 2009. Dan Balz, "After a Bruising August, Time for Obama Team to Regroup," *Washington Post*, September 2, 2009, p. A03.

7. Elizabeth Drew, "Health Care: Can Obama Swing It?," *New York Review of Books*, October 22, 2009, p. 67.

8. Theda Skocpol, *Boomerang: Health Reform and the Turn Against Government* (New York: Norton, 1997), pp.48–73; Lawrence Jacobs and Robert Shapiro, *Politicians Don't Pander: Political Manipulation and the Loss of Democratic Responsiveness* (Chicago: University of Chicago Press, 2000), Chapter 3.
9. Charles Homans, "The Party of Obama: What Are the President's Grass Roots Good For?," *Washington Monthly* (January–February, 2010).
10. Sheryl Gay Stolberg, "Taking Health Care Courtship Up Another Notch," *New York Times*, September 27, 2009.
11. His recruitment and key contributions are described in Ryan Lizza, "Peter Orszag and the Obama Budget," *The New Yorker*, May 4, 2009.
12. Interview by authors with official in Congress on January 5, 2010.
13. David M. Herszenhorn, "Fine-Tuning Led to Health Bill's $940 Billion Price Tag," *New York Times*, March 18, 2010.
14. Peter Baker, "The Limits of Rahmism." *The New York Times Magazine*, March 8, 2010.
15. Ibid.
16. Interview by authors with Executive Branch Official on January 5, 2010.
17. Interview by authors with official in Congress on January 3, 2010.
18. Quoted in Jackie Calmes, "A Policy Debate and Its Lesson: Clinton's Defeat Sways Obama's Tactics," *New York Times*, September 6, 2009.
19. Interview by authors with official in Congress on January 3, 2010.
20. Interview by authors with official in Congress on January 5, 2010.
21. Reed Abelson, "In Health Care Reform, Boons for Hospitals and Drug Makers," *New York Times,* March 22, 2010. David D. Kirkpatrick, "Lobbyists Fight Last Big Plans to Cut Health Care Costs," *New York Times,* October 10, 2009. Amy Goldstein, "Influential AMA's Support for Reform Is Far From Certain," *Washington Post,* October 16, 2009.
22. Dan Eggen, "Health-Care Effort Losing Important Player; Tauzin's Resignation from PhRMA May Add to Democrats' Problems," *Washington Post,* February 13, 2010, p. A04.
23. Interview by authors with official in Congress on January 3, 2010.
24. Reed Abelson, "In Health Care Reform, Boons for Hospitals and Drug Makers."
25. Ceci Connolly, "Ex-Foes of Health Care Reform Emerge as Supporters," *Washington Post,* March 6, 2009. Prior to becoming President and CEO of AHIP, Karen Ignagni worked as a staffer on Capitol Hill and at AFL-CIO.
26. Ibid.
27. Senator John D. Rockefeller IV during a Senate Finance Committee, September 24, 2009.

28. Reed Abelson, "President's Speech Allays Some Fears in the Health Insurance Industry," *New York Times,* September 10, 2009.
29. Steven Pearlstein, "Republicans Propagating Falsehoods in Attacks on Health-Care Reform," *The Washington Post,* August 7, 2009.
30. Reed Abelson, "In Health Care Reform, Boons for Hospitals and Drug Makers."
31. Kent Garber, "Committee Passes Baucus's $829 Billion Healthcare Bill: Republican Sen. Olympia Snowe Joined Democrats to Vote Yes on the Healthcare Reform Bill," *U.S.News,* October 13, 2009.
32. Ceci Connolly, "New Bill Would Raise Rates, Says Insurance Group; Report Issued Before Key Committee Vote," *Washington Post,* October 12, 2009.
33. Duff Wilson, "Drug Makers Raise Prices in Face of Health Care Reform," *New York Times,* November 15, 2009.
34. Ben Smith and Kenneth Vogel, "How Dems Set Stage for Corporate-Backed Health Care Campaign," *Politico,* October, 16, 2009.
35. Katharine Seelye, "Competing Ads on Health Plan Swamp Airwaves," *New York Times,* August 16, 2009."
36. Kate Zernike and Megan Thee-Brenan, "Poll Finds Tea Party Backers Wealthier and More Educated," *New York Times,* April 14, 2010.
37. Specifically, the Atlantic Philanthropies seeded the development of the Health Care for America Now (HCAN) coalition, starting in early 2008. See the retrospective overview of the foundation's role in Gara LaMarche, "A Big Bet on Advocacy Helps to Make History on Health Care," *Atlantic Currents* e-newsletter, April 4, 2010.
38. Campaign for America's Future, accessed June 23, 2010 from http://ourfuture.org/healthcare/public-health-insurance.   Jacob Hacker, "The Case for Public Plan Choice in National Health Reform: Key to Cost Control and Quality Coverage," December 16, 2008.
39. Health Care for America Now. "Who We Are," accessed May 30, 2010, from http://healthcareforamericanow.org/site/content/who_we_are/
40. Kevin Sack and Marjorie Connelly, "In Poll, Wide Support for Government-Run Health," *New York Times,* June 20, 2009. Megan Thee-Brenan, "Health Care Views Steady," *New York Times,* January 22, 2010, p. 16. Katharine Q. Seelye, "The Public's Opposition," *New York Times,* December 20, 2009, p. 20.
41. Baker, "The Limits of Rahmism."
42. Paul Krugman, "Not Enough Audacity," *New York Times,* June 26, 2009.
43. Paul Krugman, "Republican Death Trip," *New York Times,* August 14, 2009.
44. Lori Montgomery, "In Health-Care Reform, No Deficit Cure," *New York Times,* November 30, 2009.
45. President Obama, "Obama's Health Care Speech to Congress."
46. Senator Chuck Grassley, Speech on the floor of the U.S. Senate, December 10, 2009.

47. Interview by authors with official in Congress on January 5, 2010.
48. Interview by authors with official in Congress on January 5, 2010; Interview by authors with health policy advisor to Democrats in Congress and White House on February 24, 2010; Senator Chuck Grassley, Speech on the floor of the U.S. Senate, December 10, 2009.
49. Peter Dreier, "Lessons from the Health-Care Wars," *The American Prospect*, April 5, 2010.
50. Interview by authors with official in Congress on January 5, 2010.
51. Senator Chuck Grassley, Speech on the floor of the U.S. Senate, December 10, 2009; Interview by authors with official in Congress on January 5, 2010.
52. Alter, *The Promise.*
53. Jim Rutenberg and Jackie Calmes, "False 'Death Panel' Rumor Has Some Familiar Roots," *New York Times*, August 13, 2009.
54. Shailagh Murray and Lori Montgomery. "With Senate 'fixes' bill, GOP has last chance to change health-care overhaul; Debate begins on package of 'fixes' to new law," *Washington Post*, March 24, 2010.
55. In the Senate, no Republican votes ever materialized beyond Snowe's one-time vote for a committee bill; and in the House, only one Republican voted for the November bill—Representative Joseph Cao of Louisiana (elected in a bit of a fluke from a heavily Democratic district when the sitting Congressman was sent to jail for misappropriating funds).
56. McConnell quoted in Calmes, "Policy Debate."
57. Carl Hulse and Adam Nagourney, "GOP Leader Finds Weapon in Party Unity," *New York Times*, March 17, 2010.
58. Carl Hulse and Adam Nagourney, "GOP Leader Finds Weapon in Party Unity," *New York Times*, March 17, 2010.
59. Ibid.
60. Senator Chuck Grassley, Speech on the floor of the U.S. Senate, December 10, 2009.
61. Lawrence Jacobs, "1994 All Over Again? Public Opinion and Health Care," *New England Journal of Medicine*, Vol. 358, No. 18, May 1, 2008, pp. 1881–1883.
62. President Barack Obama, Speech to Congress, "Obama's Health Care Speech to Congress," September 9, 2009.
63. President Obama's speech to joint session of Congress, September 9, 2009; Reed Abelson, "President's Speech Allays Some Fears in Health Insurance Industry," *New York Times*, September 11, 2009.
64. Edmund Halsmaler and Nina Owcharenko, "The Massachusetts Approach: A New Way to Restructure State Health Insurance Markets and Public Programs," *Health Affairs*, November/December 2006; Hugh Hewitt, *A Mormon in the White House?: 10 Things Every American Should Know about Mitt Romney* (Washington, DC: Regnery Publishing).
65. Interview by authors with official in the Executive branch on January 5, 2010.

66. Obama speeches, February 24, 2009, and September 9, 2009.
67. Kaiser Family Foundation polls in 2009 and 2010 showed that, over time, Americans came to believe that their own families would be worse off because of health reform even as the uninsured, lower-income people, and others would be better off. Laura Meckler and Janet Adamy, "Obama Renews Health Push: Retooled $950 Billion Plan Aims to Get Legislation Through Over Republican Objections, *Wall Street Journal*, February 23, 2010.
68. Amy Goldstein, "Pelosi backs Medicare buy-in plan in Senate health-care deal: Speaker says Expansion has appeal, but she still prefers a public Option," *Washington Post*, December 11, 2009.
69. Representative Richard Neal (D-MA) and Judith Stein (director of Center for Medicare Advocacy) quoted in Robert Pear, "Obama Proposal to Create Medicare Panel Meets with Resistance," *New York Times*, August 14, 2009.

Chapter 3

1. Picture and caption accompanying Jessica Van Sack and Hillary Chabot, "President Obama aims to beat back Scott Brown," *Boston Herald*, January 18, 2010.
2. Fred Barnes, "The Health Care Bill Is Dead," *WeeklyStandard.com*, January 20, 2010.
3. Jessica Van Sack and Hillary Chabot, "Where Is He Now?," *Boston Herald*, March 24, 2010.
4. One of the authors, Skocpol, listens regularly to WEEI starting at 6 A.M., so these characterizations come from personally heard data.
5. Stephanie Ebbert, "Tea Party Shows Its Muscle in Bay State," *Boston Globe*, January 21, 2010, pp. A1 and A12; Casey Ross, "Financial Executives Spent Big on Brown," *Boston* Globe, February 1, 2010, pp. A1 and A5; Adam Nagourney, Jeff Zeleny, Kate Zernike, and Michael Cooper, "How the G.O.P. Captured a Seat Lost for Decades," *New York Times*, January 21, pp. A1 and A28.
6. Dan Payne, "What Voters Were Saying at the Polls," *Boston Globe*, January 27, 2010.
7. Elizabeth Drew, "Is There Life in Health Care Reform?" *New York Review of Books*, March 11, 2010, p. 49.
8. Summary of Washington Post-ABC poll results in Dan Balz and Chris Cillizza, "Senate Election in Massachusetts Could Be Harbinger for Health-Care Reform," *Washington Post*, January 19, 2010.
9. Melanie Trottman, "Union Households Gave Boost to GOP's Brown," *Wall Street Journal*, January 22, 2010, p. A3.
10. Timothy Noah, "Dream Killer," *Slate*, posted January 19, 2010.
11. The various ideas are nicely summarized in "Dream Killer," though Timothy Noah himself believed that no plan B could work if Coakley actually lost.
12. Paul Waldman argued in "Why Massachusetts Doesn't Matter," *The American Prospect*, January 19, 2010, that the "preferable" path "would be to get the bill done before Brown is sworn in."

13. "Pass the damn bill" repeatedly titled or concluded entries on Benen's blog. His fully considered call was "Project for a Healthy American Future: The Way Forward on Health Reform in 2010," *Washington Monthly*, January 25, 2010. Paul Krugman also called for the House to "Do the Right Thing" in his regular *New York Times* OpEd column published on January 22, 2010, p. A21.

14. A detailed side-by-side overview of the 2009 House and Senate bills, along with the March 2010 legislation that eventually passed, appears in "Side-By-Side Comparison of Major Health Care Reform Proposals," *Focus on Health Reform*, at the Web site of the Kaiser Family Foundation.

15. The meeting is described in the opening paragraphs of Ceci Connolly, "How Obama Revived His Health-Care Bill," *Washington Post*, March 23, 2010.

16. As quoted in ibid.

17. As quoted in ibid.

18. Shailagh Murray, Michael D. Shear, and Paul Kane, "2009 Democratic Agenda Severely Weakened by Republicans' United Opposition," *Washington Post*, January 24, 2010.

19. Drew, "Is There Life in Health Care Reform?" p. 51.

20. Reid Wilson, "Frank: Health Care Compromise: 'Dead,'" *Hotline On Call*, a blog of the *National Journal*, January 20, 2010.

21. Jonathan Karl, "Bayh Warns of 'Catastrophe' If Dems Ignore Massachusetts Senate Race Lessons," *The Note*, ABC News, January 19, 2010. Susan Davis, "Webb: No Health Care Action Until Brown Is Seated," *Washington Wire*, a blog of the *Wall Street Journal*, January 19, 2010.

22. *Wall Street* Journal, Thursday, January 21, 2010, p. A1.

23. Ibid, plus Sheryl Gay Stolberg and David M. Herszenhorn, "Obama Weighs a Paring of Goals for a Health Care Bill," *New York Times,*, January 21, 2010, pp. A1 and A26; Sam Stein, "Barack Obama, Campaign Manager: How the 2008 Playbook Passed Health Care," *Huffington Post*, first posted May 13, 2010, p. 1.

24. Sheryl Gay Stolberg, Jeff Zeleny, and Carl Hulse, "The Long Road Back." *New York Times*, March 21, 2010, pp. A1–A16.

25. Drew, "Is There Life in Health Care Reform?," pp. 50–51.

26. As quoted in ibid, p. 52.

27. Franken quoted in Ceci Connolly, "How Obama Revived His Health Care Bill."

28. Roy Edroso, "Scott Brown Wins Mass. Race, Giving GOP 41–59 Majority in the Senate," *Village Voice*, January 20, 2010.

29. John Stewart reported "As the 41st member of the minority party, Brown will now be imbued with near limitless power over financial, military, and social policy, just as our founders had intended." Ben Craw, "The Daily Show Calls It: 'Scott Brown Is Now Apparently The 45th President of These United States of America!'" TPM LiveWire, January 21, 2010.

30. Sam Stein,"Labor on Dems Who Block Health Reform: We'll 'Take Them Out,'" *Huffington Post*, March 9, 2010.

31. Scot J. Paltrow, "Wellpoint Raising Rates by Double Digits in at Least 11 States," Center for American Progress Action Fund, February 24, 2010.

32. Emily Berry, "Anthem Rate Hike Reignites Health Reform Push," posted March 1, 2010, at the Web site *amednews.com*. Berry looks back at developments throughout February. See also Christina Bellatoni, "California Insurer's Rate Hike Becomes Rallying Point for Health Care Reform," posted February 15, 2010, at *TalkingPointsMemo.com*.

33. As quoted in ibid.

34. Jonathan Alter, *The Promise: President Obama, Year One* (New York: Simon & Schuster, 2010), pp. 419–420. Ezra Klein, "Is health-care reform popular?" *Washington Post*, February 23, 2010.

35. Summary of Washington Post-ABC poll results in Dan Balz and Chris Cillizza, "Senate Election in Massachusetts Could Be Harbinger for Health-Care Reform," *Washington Post*, January 19, 2010.

36. Sam Stein, "Obama Goes to GOP Lions' Den—And Mauls the Lions," *Huffington Post*, Januray 29, 2010.

37. David M. Herszenhorn and Robert Pear, "Obama to Offer Health Bill to Ease Impasse as Bipartisan Meeting Approaches," *New York Times*, February 18, 2010. Sheryl Gay Stolberg and David M. Herszenhorn, "Obama's Health Bill Plan Largely Follows Senate Version," *New York Times*, February 22, 2010.

38. Jason M. Breslow, "Health Reform's Next Step: 23rd Use of Reconciliation?" PBS NewsHour, February 26, 2010.

39. Huma Khan, Jonathan Karl, and Z. Byron Wolf, "Health Care Bill: House Passes $938 Billion Bill, Sweeping Legislation on Its Way to Become Law," ABC News, March 21, 2010.

40. Connolly, "How Obama Revived His Health-Care Bill."

41. Shailagh Murray and Lori Montgomery, "Democrats move toward grouping health reform with student-aid bill," *Washington Post*, March 12, 2010; and Alter, *The Promise*, p. 432.

42. Alter, *The Promise*, pp.431–434; and Janet Adamy and Laura Meckler, "Vote by Vote, a Troubled Bill Was Revived," *Wall Street Journal*, Monday, March 22, 2010.

43. Dana Milbank, "Kucinich's health-care vote could be Obama's lucky charm," *Washington Post*, March 18, 2010. Christina Bellatoni, "From Holding Out to Whipping Health Care—How Dennis Kucinich Is Helping Dems Pass Reform," Talking Points Memo Web site, DC tab, March 18, 2010.

44. Alter, *The Promise*, p. 433.

45. Ibid; and David M. Herszenhorn and Robert Pear, "Democrats Rally to Obama's Call for Health Vote," *New York Times*, March 21, 2010, pp. A1 and A17.

46. Catholic differences are recounted in "Editorial: National Catholic Reporter Backs Health Bill," *National Catholic Reporter*, online edition, March 18, 2010.

47. Jake Sherman, "Randy Neugebauer: I yelled 'baby killer,'" *Politico*, March 22, 2010.

48. "Boehner: It's 'Armageddon,' Health Care Bill Will 'Ruin Our Country,'" *Fox News*, March 20, 2010.

49. Paul Kane, " 'Tea Party' protestors accused of spitting on lawmaker, using slurs," *Washington Post*, March 20, 2010.

Chapter 4

1. Lawrence R. Jacobs and Theda Skocpol, "What Americans Really Think About Health Reform," Scholars Strategy Network, May 2012. http://www.scholarsstrategynetwork.org/sites/default/files/ssn_basic_facts_jacobs_and_skocpol_on_views_on_health_reform.pdf.
2. Congressional Budget Office (CBO), "H.R. 4872, Reconciliation Act of 2010 (Final Health Care Legislation)," March 20, 2010; CBO, "Budget and Economic Outlook, 2014–2024," February 2014, Pub. No. 4869 http://cbo.gov/sites/default/files/cbofiles/attachments/45010-Outlook2014_Feb.pdf; CBO, "Updated Estimates of the Effects of the Insurance Coverage Provisions of the Affordable Care Act," April 2014, DC. Pub. No. 4930. http://www.cbo.gov/sites/default/files/
3. "What each said about the health care vote: Obama, John Boehner, Tim Kaine, Michael Steele," *Los Angeles Times*, March 22, 2010.
4. Tricia Neuman and Gretchen Jacobson, "Medicare Advantage: Take Another Look," Kaiser Family Foundation, May 7, 2014. http://kff.org/medicare/perspective/medicare-advantage-take-another-look/
5. Edwin Park, "CBO Finds Health Reform's Medicaid Expansion Is an Even Better Deal for States," Center for Budget and Policy Priorities," April 22, 2014, http://www.cbpp.org/cms/?fa=view&id=4131
6. CBO, "Updated Estimates of the Effects of the Insurance Coverage Provisions of the Affordable Care Act," April 14, 2014, https://www.cbo.gov/publication/45231.
7. Congressional Budget Office, "An Analysis of Health Insurance Premiums Under the Patient Protection and Affordable Care Act," November 30, 2009 and "Updated Estimates of the Effects of the Insurance Coverage Provisions of the Affordable Care Act." April 2014. Washington, DC. Pub. No. 4930. http://www.cbo.gov/sites/default/files/cbofiles/attachments/45231-ACA_Estimates.pdf; Kaiser Family Foundation, "2014 Employer Health Benefits Survey," September 10, 201;4http://kff.org/private-insurance/report/2014-employer-health-benefits-survey/
8. Congressional Budget Office, "H.R. 4872, Reconciliation Act of 2010 (Final Health Care Legislation)," March 20, 2010.
9. Benjamin Sommers, "Insurance Cancellations in Context: Stability of Coverage in the Nongroup Market Prior to Health Reform," Health Affairs 33 (April 2014): 700–706; Gary Claxton, Larry Levitt, Anthony Damico, and Matthew Rae, "Data Note: How Many People Have Nongroup Health Insurance?" Kaiser Family Foundation. January 3, 2014. http://kff.org/privateinsurance/issue-brief/how-many-people-havenongroup-health-insurance/;

Jonathan Cohn, "Maybe Those Obamacare Plan Cancellations Weren't As Bad As You've Heard," *New Republic*, April 24, 2014 http://www.newrepublic.com/article/117497/obamacare-cancelled-policies-study-saysimpact-was-actually-small))

10. Helen Darling (President, National Business Group on Health) quoted in Lesley Alderman, "Looking Toward Wellness Discounts," *New York Times*, April 10, 2010.

11. CBO, "Payments of Penalties for Being Uninsured Under the Affordable Care Act: 2014 Update." June 5, 2014 https://www.cbo .gov/publication/45397

12. Ezra Klein, "Is health-care reform popular?" *Washington Post*, February 23, 2010.

13. Tax Policy Center, "Medicare Tax as Proposed in H.R. 3590 (Senate Health Bill) and H.R. 4872 (Reconciliation Act of 2010) Distribution of Federal Tax Change by Cash Income Level, 2013." www. taxpolicycenter.org/numbers/displayatab.cfm?Docid=2697& DocTypeID=1; Tax Policy Center, "The American Taxpayer Relief Act of 2012 (ATRA) as Passed by the Senate; Step 2 of 7: Health Care Law Provisions; Distribution of Federal Tax Change by Cash Income Percentile, 2013," January 7, 2013, http://www .taxpolicycenter.org/numbers/displayatab.cfm?DocID=3761

14. Tax Policy Center, "Medicare Tax as Proposed in H.R. 3590 (Senate Health Bill) and H.R. 4872 (Reconciliation Act of 2010) Distribution of Federal Tax Change by Cash Income Level, 2013," www .taxpolicycenter.org/numbers/displayatab.cfm?Docid=2697& DocTypeID=1

15. Jonathan Gruber and Brigitte C. Madrian, "Health Insurance, Labor Supply, and Job Mobility: A Critical Review of the Literature," NBER Working Papers 8817, National Bureau of Economic Research, 2002; Jonathan Gruber "A Shot in the Arm: How Today's Health Care Reform Can Create Tomorrow's Entrepreneurs," *Washington Monthly*, May/June 2009; Martha Stinson, "Estimating the Relationship between Employer-Provided Health Insurance, Worker Mobility, and Wages," Paper presented at 10th International Conference on Panel Data, Berlin, July 2002.

16. John Holahan and Bowen Garrett, "How Will the Affordable Care Act Affect Jobs?" March 2011. Urban Institute; Derek Thompson, "2014: The Best Year for Job Creation This Century," The Atlantic. October 3, 2014. http://www.theatlantic.com/business/archive/ 2014/10/jobs-day-unemployment-rate-lowest-since-july-2008/ 381083/

17. CBO, "The Budget and Economic Outlook: 2014 to 2024." February 2014. http://cbo.gov/sites/default/files/cbofiles/attachments/45010-Outlook2014_Feb.pdf.

18. Affordable Care was a key factor in the sharp slowdown in health inflation as were other factors—most notably, the economic slowdown. But costs have remained below historic rates of growth well after the economy expanded. CBO, "Updated Estimates of the

Effects of the Insurance Coverage Provisions of the Affordable Care Act." April 2014. Washington, DC. Pub. No. 4930. http://www .cbo.gov/sites/default/files/cbofiles/attachments/45231-ACA_ Estimates.pdf ; Doug Elmendorf, "Estimating the Budgetary Effects of the Affordable Care Act," June 17, 2014, https://www.cbo.gov/ publication/45447.

19. The Commonwealth Fund. "The Affordable Care Act's Payment and Delivery System Reforms: A Progress Report at Five Years." May 7, 2015. http://www.commonwealthfund.org/publications/ issue-briefs/2015/may/aca-payment-and-delivery-system-reforms-at-5-years (accessed July 23, 2015).

20. Medicare's administrators did pause the planned Medicare Advantage reductions for 2016 owing to increased spending in the traditional Medicare program. Centers for Medicare and Medicaid Services. "Fact Sheet: Moving Medicare Advantage and Part D Forward." April 6, 2015. http://www.cms.gov/Newsroom/Media ReleaseDatabase/Fact-sheets/2015-Fact-sheets-items/2015-04-06 .html (accessed July 23, 2015).

21. Jonathan Gruber (health economist at Massachusetts Institute of Technology) quoted in Karen Tumulty, Kate Pickert with Alice Part, "What Will It Cost?" *Time*, March 25, 2010.

22 The Commission, which is officially titled the Independent Payment Advisory Board, is composed of experts and stakeholders who are appointed by the president, need Senate confirmation, and serve six-year terms.

23. Merrill Goozner, "Smaller Payouts, Lower Fees Slow Medicare Spending." *The Fiscal Times*, April 25, 2012.

24. John Wennberg and Alan Gittelsohn, 'Variations in Medical Care among Small Areas," *Scientific American*, Vol. 246, No 4, April 1982, pp.120–134; W. Pete Welch, Mark E. Miller, H. Gilbert Welch, Elliott S. Fisher, and John E. Wennberg, "Geographic Variation in Expenditures for Physicians' Services in the United States," *New England Journal of Medicine*, Vol. 328, No. 9, March 4, 1993, pp. 621–627.

Chapter 5

1. Legislature of the State of Idaho, Sixtieth Legislature, Second Regular Session 2010, House Bill No. 391, http://www.legislature .idaho.gov/legislation/2010/H0391.pdf.

2. Joel Ario and Lawrence Jacobs, "In the Wake of the Supreme Court Decision Over the Affordable Care Act, Many Stakeholders Still Support Health Reform," *Health Affairs*, Web Publication, July 11, 2012.

3. Reed Abelson, "A Scrappy Insurer Wrestles with Reform," *New York Times*, May 16, 2010.

4. Christopher Jennings, "Implementation and Legacy of Health Care Reform," *New England Journal of Medicine*, April 24, 2010.

5. Interview by authors with Congressional official on January 5, 2010.

6. Jason Millman, "Jawboning by HHS doesn't scare insurers," *Politico*, May 8, 2012.

7. The Obama administration reversed its proposals for 2.3 percent cut for Medicare Advantage plans in 2014 (as the ACA anticipated) into a 3.3 percent increase; its proposed 1.9 percent reduction for 2015 payments was flipped to a 0.4 percent increase. A similar decision increased (rather than cut) rates by 1.25% for 2016. Caroline Humer, "Government payments for Medicare Advantage plans to rise in 2016." Reuters, April 6, 2015. http://www.reuters.com/article/2015/04/06/us-usa-healthcare-medicare-idUSKBN0MX1E120150406; Jason Millman, "Medicare Reversed Payment Cuts, and Not Many Are Happy about It," Washington Post Wonkblog, April 14, 2014 http://www.washingtonpost.com/blogs/wonkblog/wp/2014/04/14/medicarereversed-payment-cuts-and-not-many-are-happyabout-it//?print51.

8. Robert Pear, "Health Insurance Companies Try to Shape Rules," New York Times, May 16, 2010; Brianna Ehley, "How An Obamacare Tweak Could Save Insurers Millions," Fiscal Times, July 17, 2014 http://www.thefiscaltimes.com/Articles/2014/07/17/How-Obamacare-Tweak-Could-Save-Insurers-Millions#sthash.VLxi1nOs.dpuf

9. Ibid.

10. Robert Pear, "Obama Health Team Turns to Carrying Out Law."

11. F. Schouten, "Health Industry Invests in States," *USA Today*, April 2, 2010, p. A1. Public advocates have organized in some states to challenge business and professional associations. Timothy Callaghan and Lawrence R. Jacobs, "The Interest Group Battle Over Medicaid Expansion: The Surprising Impact of Public Advocates," *American Journal of Public Health*, Forthcoming.

12. Paul N. Van de Water, "Excise Tax on Medical Devices Should Not Be Repealed: Industry Lobbyists Distort Tax's Impact," Center for Budget Priority and Policy," October 2, 2013, http://www.cbpp.org/cms/?fa=view&id=3684; Ron Way, "Repealing device tax? Unnecessary," *Star Tribune*, November 16, 2014 http://www.startribune.com/opinion/commentaries/282773011.html.

13. Edwin Park, "CBO Finds Health Reform's Medicaid Expansion Is an Even Better Deal for States," Center for Budget and Policy Priorities," April 22, 2014, http://www.cbpp.org/cms/?fa=view&id=413.

14. Kaiser Family Foundation, "Consumer Oriented and Operated Plan (CO-OP) Loans Awarded," http://kff.org/health-reform/state-indicator/co-op-loans/; National Alliance of State Health CO-Ops, "Over 400,000 people now enrolled in CO-OP health insurance plans," April 24, 2014, http://nashco.org/over-400000-people-now-enrolled-in-co-op-health-insurance-plans/ However, Congressional Republicans pressured Democrats in 2012 to reduce spending on non-profit cooperatives from $6 billion to $3.4 billion, as part of the "fiscal-cliff" negotiations. Those budget cuts have reduced federal funding for new efforts.

15. Lawrence R. Jacobs and Theda Skocpol, "Progressive Federalism and the Contested Implementation of Obama's Health Reform," *The Politics of Major Policy Reform*, edited by Jeffrey Jenkins and Sidney Milkis, Cambridge, UK: Cambridge University Press, 2014; Timothy Callaghan and Lawrence R. Jacobs, "Process Learning and the Implementation of Medicaid Reform," *Publius: The Journal of Federalism* 44 (Fall 2014): 541–563.

16. Robert Myers, "How bad were the original actuarial estimates for Medicare's hospital insurance program?" *The Actuary*, February 1994; Lawrence Jacobs, *The Health of Nations: The Making of the American Medicare Act of 1965 and the British National Health Service Act of 1946* (Ithaca, NY.: Cornell University Press, 1993).

17. The federal government picks up all the costs of individuals who first become eligible for newly expanded Medicaid from 2014 to 2016. Then the share paid by states gradually increases to 10% by 2020—while states that, as of now, already offer expanded coverage to the poor will enjoy increases in federal support.

18. Senator Alexander quoted in "Questioning the Cost of Health Care Overhaul," *New York Times*, April 3, 2010; Kim Belshe quoted in Michael Luo, "Some States Find Burdens in Health Law," *New York Times*, March 27, 2010.

19. Robert Berenson, Paul Ginsburg, Jon Christianson, and Tracy Yee, "The Growing Power of Some Providers to Win Steep Payment Increases from Insurers Suggests Policy Remedies May Be Needed," *Health Affairs* 31(May 2012): 973–81.

20. James R. Horney and Paul N. Van de Water, "House-Passed and Senate Health Bills Reduce Deficit," *Report of Center of Budget and Policy Priorities*, December 4, 2009; Ezra Klein, "Can We Control Costs without Congress?" *Washington Post*, March, 26, 2010; Ezra Klein, "Can Congress Cut Medicare Costs?" *Washington Post* online, December 4, 2009.

21. Part of the misinformation campaign is the misleading charge—as made by Republican Congressman Jim Gerlach and repeated by *New York Times* columnist David Brooks—that the new legislation "calls for the American people to spend 10 years paying for six years of benefits." The reality, as documented by the CBO, is that little or no money is spent or raised in the first three years of the program, and significant revenues are generated in the final five or six years of the first decade. Gerlach quoted in "Questioning the Cost of Health Care Overhaul," *New York Times*, April 3, 2010. See also Brooks, "The Emotion of Reform," *New York Times*, March 8, 2010; Congressional Budget Office, "Director's Blog," April 12, 2010; and Ezra Klein, "The Affordable Care Act Does Not have 10 years of taxes for six years of spending," *Washington Post* Online, April 12, 2010.

22. Center for Health Information and Analysis, "Annual Report on the Performance of the Massachusetts Health Care System," September 2014, http://ow.ly/H8ZhP.

23. Quoted in Jackie Calmes, "After Health Care Passage, Obama Pushes to Get It Rolling," *New York Times*, April 18, 2010.

24. The official Republican stance going into the fall 2010 elections was explained in Molly K. Hooper, "GOP Moves to Repeal Healthcare Law," *The Hill*, June 2, 2010.

25. Richard Himelfarb, *Catastrophic Politics: The Rise and Fall of the Medicare Catastrophic Coverage Act of 1988* (University Park: University of Pennsylvania Press, 1995).

26. Hooper, "GOP Moves to Repeal Healthcare Law"; Molly K. Hooper, "Internal Grumbling Over Republican Healthcare Message Intensifies," *The Hill*, April 8, 2010; B. Reisinger, "Corker: Health Reform Won't Be Repealed," *Nashville Business Journal*, April 1, 2010; James Capretta and Robert Moffit, "How to Replace Obamacare," *National Affairs* 11 (Spring 2012).

27 J. Young, "AARP, Dems Lobby Older Voters on Healthcare Law before Midterms," *The Hill*, April 8, 2010; Sarah Wheaton, "Medicare in the 2014 campaign: New ads, old messages," Politico, November 2, 2014 http://www.politico.com/story/2014/11/medicare-in-the-2014-campaign-new-ads-old-messages-112391.html.

28. Lloyd Free and Hadley Cantril, *The Political Beliefs of Americans* (New Brunswick, NJ: Rutgers University Press, 1967); Benjamin Page and Lawrence Jacobs, *Class War? What Americans Really Think about Economic Inequality* (Chicago: University of Chicago Press, 2009).

29. Kaiser Family Foundation Tracking Polls. http://www.kff.org/kaiserpolls/trackingpoll.cfm

30. See Lawrence R. Jacobs and Theda Skocpol, *Inequality and American Democracy: What We Know and What We Need to Learn* (New York: Russell Sage Foundation, 2005); and Larry M. Bartels, *Unequal Democracy: The Political Economy of the New Gilded Age* (Princeton, NJ: Princeton University Press, and New York: Russell Sage Foundation, 2008).

31. Andrea Louise Campbell, *How Policies Make Citizens* (Princeton, NJ: Princeton University Press, 2003).

INDEX